FORWARD

In the salt of tears, a seed takes root through the cracks of a broken world. It pushes and grows; a bud breaks through thorns, opening petals.

The rose's fragrance fills the air. Dandelions grow beside them, their petals flying in the wind wild, beautiful, and bold.

Dandelion seeds scatter in fertile soil, life renewing again and again. More life even in struggle. Always more to life than the struggle.

-N.B. Brignoni

PREFACE

"Prepare to be reminded of the special resilience found only in the wildest flowers with their rare count of petals. Within these pages, you'll discover more than just poems; you'll meet a little warrior of a flower, thriving and blooming petal by petal. To those walking a similar path, I hope you find comfort and companionship in these words. To those unfamiliar with this world, I invite you to open your heart to a different kind of beauty. Thank you for joining me on this poetic exploration of life's most important lessons, taught by the smallest of teachers my beautiful children."

- N.B. Brignoni

DEDICATION

To my Wolf-Hirschhorn warrior my little girl who taught me so much since you were a seed in my belly blooming beautifully. My warrior, your resilience fuels me every day. I watch your ability in therapy sessions to fall and rise again. This resilent sight replays in my my mind and strengthens my heart and soul by the day.

I share your story so that other flowers may remember: you have bloomed, petal by petal, despite the harshest weather. You stand tall as a beautiful sunzilla sunflower, even with missing petals perfect as you bloom.

You've taught me so much, like strength and perfection comes in many forms. Sometimes, we must set aside the science to honorably love all flowers, flawless as they are missing petals or added doesn't change their beauty.

Bloom boldly, not just to my daughters but to all flowers; you all belong here, and you always will. This world is a garden awaiting your one-of-a-kind beauty. Go, dare to bloom in the storm they think you can't withstand but little do they know you can and you will.

-N.B. Brignoni

LEGAL DISCLAIMER

The content of this book, The Missing Petals on Chromosome Four, is intended for informational and artistic purposes only. It reflects the personal experiences, opinions, and creative expressions of the author and should not be interpreted as medical advice, diagnosis, or treatment. While the author and publisher have made every effort to ensure the accuracy and completeness of the information presented, we make no representations or warranties of any kind, express or implied, regarding the completeness, accuracy, reliability, suitability, or availability of the information, products, services, or related graphics. Any reliance placed on such information is strictly at your own risk. The author and publisher disclaim any liability for any direct, indirect, incidental, consequential, or other damages resulting from the use or inability to use the information contained in this book. Medical information is based on the author's personal experience and understanding at the time of writing. As medical knowledge and best practices evolve, always consult qualified healthcare professionals for advice, diagnosis, or treatment." "Names, characters, places, and incidents are either products of the author's imagination or are used fictitiously. Any resemblance to actual persons, living or dead, events, or locales is purely coincidental. The reference to Pinocchio's growing nose in this poetry collection is used metaphorically and represents a transformative, artistic interpretation of the concept. This usage is considered fair use under 17 U.S.C. § 107. The author does not claim ownership of the Pinocchio character or story, which is in the public domain in some jurisdictions but may still be under

COPYRIGHT

Cover Design: N.B. Brignoni

Illustrations: N.B. Brignoni and Ampi Esguerra
Printed in the United States of America

CHAPTER 1 THE SEED

KISSED BY THE SUN

This chapter delves into the early stages of diagnosis and the initial shock that comes with discovering my child's medical condition.

Although, I see it in my head is a lot different from reality. I see something else. I see a garden of love, a rare sunzilla sunflower my daughter how she blooms in my belly. with a flame at its center where the nectar is supposed to lie. But what makes this sunflower truly unique isn't just its fiery core. You don't need to look closely to notice the gaps where petals should be there are flames.

And still, this sunflower remains beautiful, even with its missing parts. The gaps, however, are signs of a condition that challenges this rare sunflower and its flame. Yet, this beautiful flower won't face its struggle alone. Soon, you will understand what the missing petals signify and how they confront the sunflower.

This chapter delves into the early stages of diagnosis—the symptoms and the initial shock of discovering my child's condition. The poems within often use free verse, forgoing formal grammar, to capture the raw, chaotic emotions of that time.

Occasionally, a haiku appears to offer moments of clarity. You'll soon discover how my family and I strive to find hope when the world seems determined to tear it away. The pages featuring italicized poetry indicate the presence of both poems and art. In this chapter, the art visually represents a seed nestled within my womb. Let the italicized words guide your gaze as you absorb the canvas.

The rest of the chapters I would like the poems to speak for themselves.

P.S. readers there will be light again despite the clouds you may see in early on chapters.

-n.b. brignoni

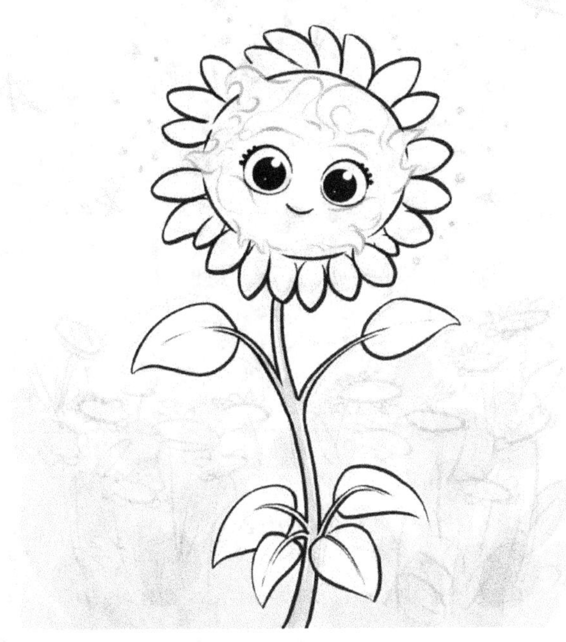

a flower with missing petals

still blooms

beauty in its own unicorn way

-n.b. brignoni

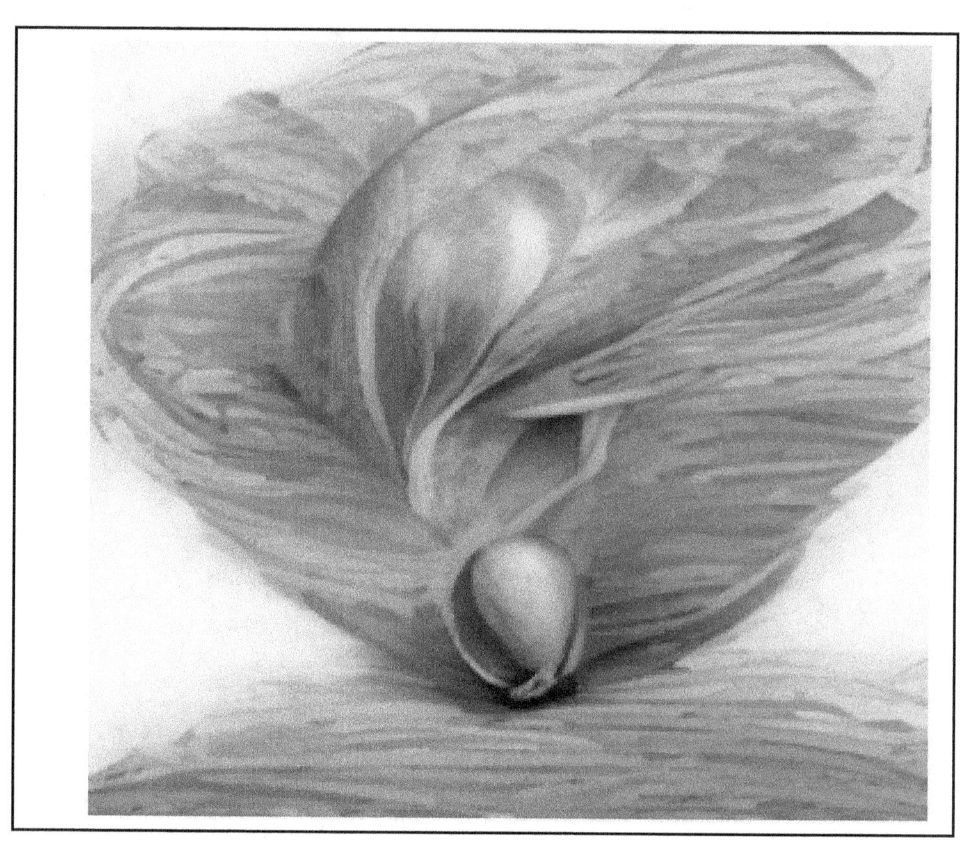

A womb's

seed—planted, in the medical field

they say a fetus, but I call it

human magic.

Because

isn't it?

-N.B. Brignoni

The Special Seed Ready to Bloom

Words carved from open wounds, bloody and bare, vulnerable pieces of her journal shed like a snake's skin. A mother, fueled by love and fear, shares her daughter's story through pages of her journal and in the power of poetry.

Raw pain and joy intertwined here, may a seedling of words take root and sprout hopeful compassion in the rich soil of your heart dear reader.

May they bloom into a garden of understanding and love for flowers with missing petals.

-N.B. Brignoni

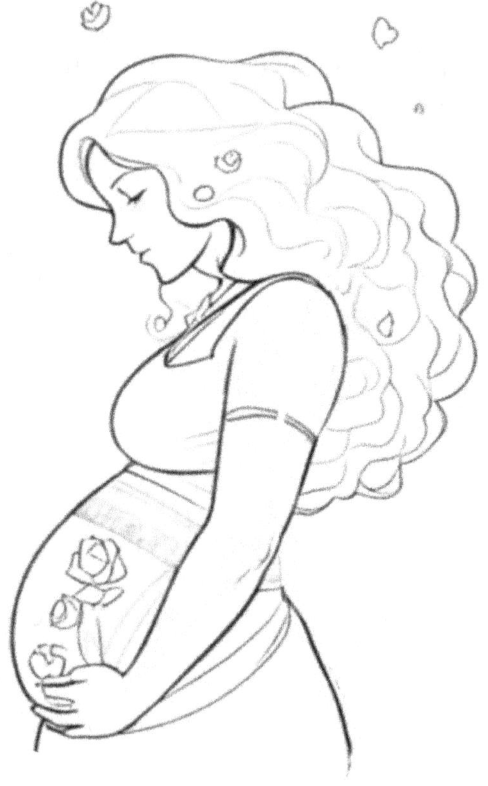

Sometimes seeds sprout differently in the womb. In some cases,
sometimes petals are fallen, and a mother's heart fills with
worry. But wait until you see the beauty in the bloom.
                                                    - N.B. Brignoni

Bloom In The Desert

My placenta, a broken organ, unable to
nourish you, my little seed.

Obstetrician's words: "Not growing enough,
amniotic fluid dangerously low."

Fear took root like a cold vine twisting
around my ribs after the cold spread of gel,
the probing wand searching for the sound of
your heartbeat while all I could hear were
the ultrasound waves crashing against my
aching heart.

This skin, once battling body dysmorphia,
now loathes every curve for failing to
nurture your growth.

Each protein-packed bite, a prayer for your
weight. Three gallons of water a day— each
sip a desperate flood, begging every drop to
reach you.

My skin stretched, but my body remained
your dry land when you needed a downpour.

Yet, my body failed.

They pulled you out early, three pounds too
small for this world.

But, my little seedling, with so little water,
you bloomed, reaching for the sun, strongest
even then.

"IUGR baby," they said— a name that never
fit.

You were a tiny warrior, with Athena's godly
strength in your small limbs— a name far
more fitting for my miracle baby.

-N.B. Brignoni

the box i made my home

love at first sight

is real

i knew this

the moment

you emerged

from the womb

our first meeting

your warm cheeks

pressed against mine

but then they ripped you

from my arms

said three pounds

was too small

and your fragile body

needed extra help

so they placed you

in a plastic box

your new home

before your newborn scent
could even become mine

as they wheeled you away
from my sight

i lay empty
unaccustomed
to being
without you

my body ached for you
and i felt
so blue

completely
and utterly lost
with you in the nicu

for thirty-five weeks
and three days

you were attached
to my body
like a limb
next to my beating heart

so being

without you

could never feel right

but even

when you were rooms away

i couldn't escape

your warmth on my cheeks

and chest lingering like you never left

i knew home

wouldn't feel sweet

until you

were right there

with me

the hospital

discharged me

before you

so it hurt

to pack my

hospital bag

when i knew
i wasn't leaving
without you
in my arms

-n.b. brignoni

second neonatal unit visit

when i saw you

the second time around

sleeping with

a radiant warmer

over your head

i wanted

to be that box

so badly

keeping you warm

while providing oxygen

instead of intravenous lines

and endotracheal tubes

up your nose

why did my body fail you

both inside the womb and out?

for a while

i wasn't well

attempting to process this news

but then

the nicu nurses

let me hold you

and i couldn't help it

a change in mood

shocked me

something

so perfect came out of me

transforming sadness

into an overwhelming

sense of happiness

as i witnessed your first smile

in your sleep

another transformation occurred

suddenly life was worth living even more

i am strong now

we are stronger together

i had to leave the unit

but every day i showed up for morning

rounds

and then i stayed for hours

until the nurses told me to shower

to care for myself so i could care for you

better

i listened anything for you

but even when i left

i couldn't stay away

i had to visit every night

i loved you

from the neonatal box

i made it my new home

until they finally said it

you graduated

from the neonatal unit

so long as you saw

the kidney specialist the day after

this was the first sign

something wasn't right

-n.b. brignoni

the imprinted box that held my heart

i ached
to be
your plastic box

my arms
its walls

my breath
a soft breeze
on your skin

my breast
your sustenance
no beeping machines
no tubes
no wires

just you
and me safe
rocking on a comfy chair

but i couldn't
make this daydream

come true

my tear-streaked

handprint

on the plastic box

is the closest

i'll get

for now

-n.b. brignoni

CHAPTER 2: HOME SWEET HOME IN COVID'S BUBBLE

face masked flowers

you were

a COVID infant

born

in the season

of face masks

in the heart

of lockdown

our world

shrank

to four walls

a computer screen

our window

to a world

we couldn't touch

at four months old

you had a virtual checkup

the doctor mentioned delays

as i opened the curtains

letting sunlight in

oblivious to doctor's concerns

as a first-time parent
i didn't grasp
the concept of "normal"

unmet milestones
weren't a worry

the doctor's alarm
went unheard

a red flag flew
over my head

but i was too busy
learning the ropes
of parenthood during lockdown

while referrals were written
therapists
assigned

this virtual visit
didn't scare me like it should've

you'd bloom

in your own time
i thought

you and i unaware
of the world outside

screaming "normal"
and "not"

when we ventured out
it was a world
of social distance

of muted sneezes
in public places

a world
that had lost its grip
on "normal" too

-n.b. brignoni

Shapeshifts & smiles

In the COVID bubble you rolled over three months late; it didn't matter to me. I wasn't keeping track of time but your doctor's did.

We celebrated each milestone late or on time like it was normal, with claps and a bubble party at home a celebration of a milestone met in isolation.

As the COVID curfew lifted. I was excited to focus on new dventures with you.

I'd start to plan the places we'd go: the beach, zoo, or playground.

Little did I know the world would later shapeshift in a different way. Our plans would defer.

Because a storm was coming with a change in our world that no parent could ever prepare their child for nor would they wish for them to endure such a storm.

-n.b. brignoni

First Therapy Arena

Months of virtual therapy confined us to our living room corner, a stage set with pillows, mats, and rattles.

You smile at your physical therapist a friendly voice on a screen. She guides my hands, teaching me the lessons of rolling, sitting, and grasping.

We learned together, celebrating tiny wins in a world on pause. I became your guide, your cheerleader, your physical therapist.

You rolled over three months late, celebrated with claps and a bubble party a milestone met in isolation.

Then, a thaw. The COVID curfew lifted, and the world creaked open its doors. Restaurants buzzed, and therapy centers welcomed tiny masked faces.

And you, eleven months old, blossomed in human touch, your laughter echoing through long hallways.

Even masked smiles formed a rainbow bridge over the terror of another seizure.

My days as your therapist were over; I could focus on the fun stuff you loved. Or so I thought.

-n.b brignoni

No Empty Boxes

Little one, no need to worry.
In my eyes you'll always be more than
enough.

Maybe there are empty boxes on the world's
list of normal. As the doctor's scratch their
heads in confusion.

You a beautiful medical mystery.

And while they count the things you have yet
to achieve. Just know you leave no empty
boxes in my heart's booklet of milestones.

Each and every one you meet them all.

Every check is marked in my heart's list the
only ones that truly count.

I love you baby further than the moon and
back.

-N.B. Brignoni

neonatal notes

primitive reflex

absent

a misfire

of neurons

a dysfunction

in the brain

and nervous system

tiny fingers

a fumbled grasp

nurses note

where was

your palmar reflex?

oh the things we did not know

no tiny toes that wiggle wide

nurses note

where was

your plantar reflex?

oh the things we did not know

knees drawn but no tense frame no fists

clenched

nurses note

where was

your moro reflex?

oh the things we did not know

a step but your leg stayed earthbound

nurses note

where was

your stepping reflex?

nurses note

oh the things we did not know

nurses notes

become silent alarms

screeches in my heart

oh the signs i missed

in a world masked

and six feet apart

-n.b. brignoni

lessons i thought you'd learn later

life is unfair

i already knew

but for you

i wished it

weren't true

a lesson taught

seven days

before your first birthday

all i wanted

was your peaceful rest

after a successful therapy session

but right after

physical therapy

a tonic-clonic seizure

seized your body

your small limbs shook

your eyes rolled back

staring blank at the ceiling

i screamed your name

no response

i scooped you

from your chair

you were an earthquake

in my arms

i placed you on your side

protected

your airway

my heart hammered against my ribs

each beat my heart ready

to burst through my chest

like open heart surgery with no saving

remedy

as your lips turned blue

with a shaking i'd never seen

i had thought
you were gone
before you
could even
turn one.

-n.b. brignoni

you were the earthquake in my arms

i almost died

on the dining

room floor

watching

your lips

turn blue

my heart

rate through

the roof

helplessly

lying there

staring at you shake

i couldn't

save

you.
 my lips almost
 changed colors
 too.

-n.b. brignoni

first scary seizure and its lessons

i'll never forget

the scariest day

of my life

the silence

after your seizure

passed was deafening

still no response

your body shaking your eyes rested

not even the ambulance sirens

could be heard

a fear and an anxiety

i'd never known

before not knowing

how to help

but in that moment

of you coming

back from the seizure

as the medics barge through the door

i also knew

i would do anything

to protect you

to fight for you

to study how to be your shield

against a silent science

in your brains neurons

no matter the cost

i would do everything

in my power

   to draw away from fearful apprehension

and solely be ready

to protect and love you

stirring clear of the dark clouds

those thoughts of the world being unfair

to you, my little one

i need to let them go

because they leave me

sad and mad at the world

who still blessed me with you

the greatest gift i could ever hold and love
forever.

-n.b. brignoni

Visiting Hours

The chill of the children's hospital room
raises goosebumps on my arms.

As I hold you tightly on a hospital bed bare of
mural art and cheerful sounds.

Yet, your father's face at the door with a loud
knock— and how he makes you smile— it
creates a heartwarming fire that melts the
icicles of fear on my soul.

The only source of warmth that could for
now.

-n.b. brignoni

CHAPTER 3: THE RED FLAGS VINES CROSSING MY THROAT IN THE MIX OF A HURRICANE

First month home

I know love; I know your father's love

and many more forms.

But the love of your child

it is something else.

It's something

out of this world.

It is living a dream

in real-time.

-N.B. Brignoni

Do you know love?

I thought I knew love in all its glorious forms: love of my mother, love of my father, love of my basketball coaches, love of my best friend, love of my teachers, love of my family, love of my first romantic partner, love of my job, love of my home.

But you, my first-born—the plot twist of my definition of love.

I never could imagine a bond so rich, a feeling that hits entirely different from what I once knew of love before.

So perhaps, I never truly knew love all the way until you came along.

-N.B. Brignoni

The Carousel of Specialists

The NICU found something in your blood: kidneys, too small, with high creatinine levels, unable to filter potassium.

Months pass; you're almost two now.

As time flies, so do the "why?" questions. No reflexes? No steps, no words? Developmental delays? I dreamt you'd walk, you'd talk.

They said, "Don't rush it. Once they start, they don't stop." I believed them.

But hope is an eggshell cracking on the MRI and ultrasounds.

Each test revealing underdeveloped organs, new diagnoses: Stage 3 Chronic Kidney Disease, Corpus Callosum Dysgenesis.

And now we await neurology results a reminder of memory stuck unconsciously on replay: a tonic seizure wrecking your infant body. Unresponsive eyes.

The left arm shakes, then the right, then your whole body—an earthquake in my chest while my arms shake with your body.

As I watched your lips turn blue, screaming responses to the 911-dispatcher's questions.

I tried to shut out the darkness, but optimism faded when I saw your body post-seizure, tired on a hospital bed not a crib it dwarfed your tiny frame.

On cold sheets, I tried to warm you with my hands, like trying to start a campfire with two slim sticks.

The nurse gently stopped me, saying not to worry with an empathetic smile. "I have a blanket warmer," she said, slowly taking the sheets from my hands as if they were a grenade.

But I know she saw the fire in my hands, the wildfire that spread from my heart to my sweaty palms.

Yet still, the doctors are at a lost for answers.

They're stumped you're a puzzle unsolved. They say if you have one more seizure, maybe it's epilepsy.

This one was a free pass, but one more could be a red flag. They can't be sure too many illnesses, all at once. So, they send us to a neurologist for testing.

After this frightful day, I knew something wasn't right—red flags now felt like bullets to my lungs.

And for months, we're passed like a hot potato through a carousel of specialists, each horse a doctor from every organ's field.

Lost in the dizzying spin, a ride with no joy only fear.

N.B. Brignoni

the climb at rock bottom

we stand

on the rocks

thrown from the top

you and i, fall at our feet

and the view of the mountaintop

above us daunting from below

what will medical results show

when we've already made it

to the bottom trying to climb

back up to feel the sun on our face

-n.b. brignoni

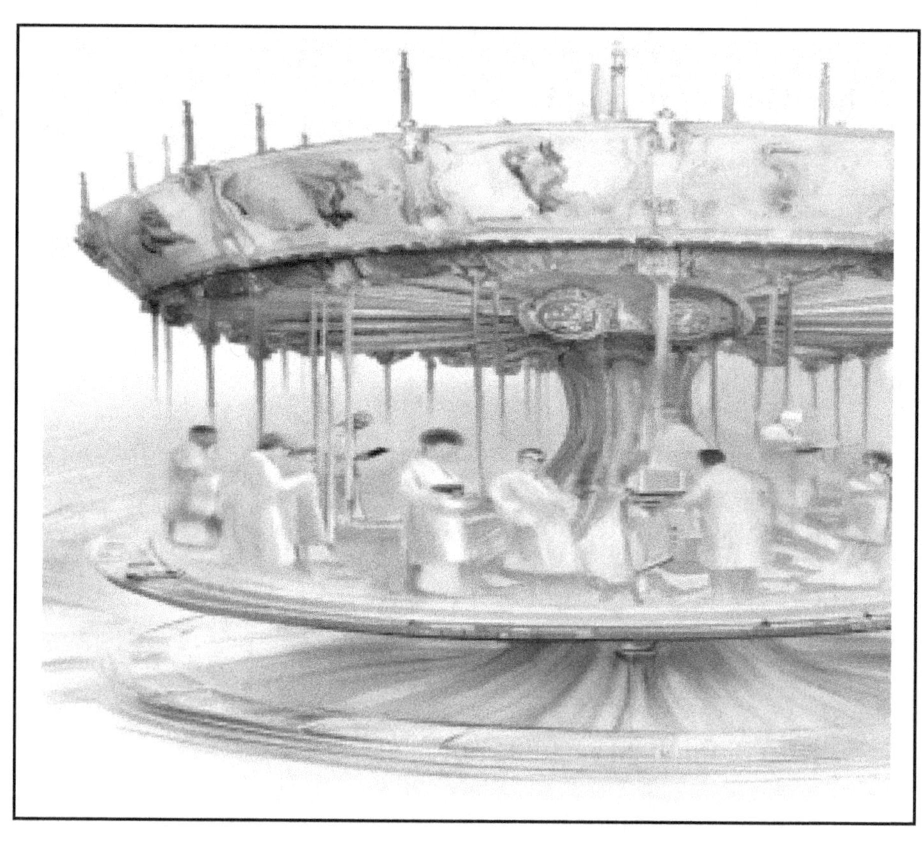

Here is a carousel
that no child
should ever ride
yet my little one
has been on it
for too long
every spin
my heart cracks
more and more.

-N.B. Brignoni

When the World Turned to Ice

One last horse.

The genetics specialist.

I wasn't worried about this one because, genetically, in you I couldn't spot a sickness.

You had been picture-perfect; plus the NICU ran its blood tests, genes tested and all had been well.

I thought we'd jump off the ride with joy, but she finds the roots—a tangled vine connected to all the red flags.

And then, as she spots an illness, the carousel and everything around it turns to ice.

Except you were the sun, ready to melt this icy world.

-N.B. Brignoni

When My Heart Turns To Ashes

The doctor's call, a confident voice: "We have the answers. To every question, every medical complication, since the day you were pregnant. We found the reason. But you must come in," she says.

"You and the father, could you come in to see us? An opening in three hours" Panic makes my heart rate climb as I asked, "could you tell me now is it bad?"

Silence on the line, that scared me even more.

She could only give me an invitation, a promise to answer every question in person at my arrival.

The thirty-minute drive, a blur of tears, and a knot in my stomach.

Baby girl, they did. They found the answers we spent almost two years searching for it was a rare chromosomal disorder.

She called it Wolf-Hirschhorn Syndrome.

Fifty-four missing genes on chromosome four, de novo evolved on their own not inherited.

Genetic tests confirm. "There is no cure," they say as my heart breaks a million pieces on the floor.

The pain of this truth hits differently, not the familiar heartbreak, the slow crumbling.

This pain is a wildfire of a savage beast, igniting the fragments of my heart of what was left.

A fire in my chest, no air in my lungs.

I try to gather the ashes of my heart, but they slip through my fingers, leaving only emptiness.

My sweat prickles my skin.

As the doctor hesitates, to answer your father's question about what this meant for your future.

In the silence we watched the doctor closely she presses her lips together, gulped her saliva.

What does it mean i had asked but couldn't say in my tears if you, my beautiful bloom were missing fifty-four petals on chromosome four.

-N.B. Brignoni

Your Father's Strong Smile

I tried to be strong, walking into that room

after the call, the urgent summons.

But I crumbled.

Couldn't hold it together— not on the drive,
not in the sterile white doctors office.

Your father, he stood tall.

Unbroken, he was whole.

He held you close, while my knees buckled

in the room's corner, swallowing the tissue
box.

Meanwhile, your nose nuzzled his.

His smile, a shield, hiding the cracks

in his own heart,

while shielding your eyes

from my broken shell

He distracted you, an umbrella against my fizzling voice and the downpour from my eyes.

I failed you.

I was the eye of the storm, the hurricane growing in category levels.

My tears flooding the room.

I should've been stronger, but I couldn't hide the pain, nor could I calm the storm of questions raging within me.

Your father, much like you, amazes me with his strength.

He held you with a stitched smile.

I don't understand how his stitches didn't come apart, as if the doctor didn't break our hearts. Then run them over with a big yellow bus.

"Chromosome four, missing parts. Your daughter may never walk or talk, no chance at games of chess. I am a doctor; I can't play that myself." She chuckled as if it were okay to compare and joke in a sensitive time.

Your future, the doctor had written, like she had a crystal ball, revealing a life story low-spirited.

Meanwhile, I was a Category 5 hurricane, needing an extra tissue box.

Your father kept it together, even though those words crushed us both.

He wouldn't let the darkness in, not while you were in his arms.

And I don't know how he did it, made you laugh till you cried.

Your father, a mountain against the volcanic eruption, stood tall with lava dripping on his skin, not a single rock breached.

You are so strong like him, not me.

The supermom cape, had got tattered and
torn, lost in the hurricane winds.

-N.B. Brignoni

the garden we rebuild

i take your hand

with a smile

ready to walk

and let go of what i know

through the path of thorns and blooms

praying I can take every prick that comes

instead of you so you can bloom in this unknown

garden all of us can't wait for you to grow.

-n.b. brignoni

i'm no superhero

but i know

if i have to be

strong for someone

it'll be

for you

my little one

-n.b. brignoni

For You, Pinky Promises

I will learn to heal

and to be stronger

for you

For you

are

my little warrior

my guiding star

my moon

and there is nothing

in this world

I wouldn't learn

to do

for you

-n.b. brignoni

93 Billion Light-Years

off the carousel,
words still tying knots
in the pit of my stomach.
frozen,
in a world of maybes.

but then,
i see you,
a belly laugh erupting,
shared with your dad.

your strength,
a guiding star,
illuminating the path
through the Wolf-Hirschhorn maze.

in the future's uncertainty,
one thing is certain:
you'll be so loved,
no matter what may come.

and my love for you,
unmoved,
even if the maybes are true.

i'd love you
not just to the moon and back,
but from here
to the 93 billion light-years
in the universe
and back again.

my sunflower,
glowing,
always beautiful.

missing petals
only add
to your perfect picture.

i capture this moment,
you and your father,
forever tattooed on my heart.

the only thing
that ever mattered
from the start.

-N.B. Brignoni

True Warrior, you

Random seizures
and low functioning organs
this is the heartless science
I can't control
can't fix

My mind circles,
a dizzy, dark spiral.

It's breaking my heart.

It hurts.
It hurts.

No cure.

Sadness mixed into fear,
overwhelmed by the gambles
of threat.

But you, Athena,
a true warrior,
face each day
with a strength
I can only dream of.

- N.B. Brignoni

Mom's Heart Breaking Repeatedly

Radio calls,
one-year-old girl,
body seizing.

Mom,
in the background,
screams,
"no
no
not you
not my baby."

She questions reality.

Why this
illness too?
Why this
burden for a baby?

She begs
to take her
instead,
to carry it all,

the illnesses
in her
daughter's body.

She longs for playpen giggles,
for carefree days,
a childhood untouched by seizures.

But instead,
her little one
carries burdens,
the weight of every
sea
on
earth.

Yet, in her tears,
she dispenses emergency medicine,
her daughter's way
back to consciousness.

Her little girl
wakes in a blur
of salty kisses and hugs
on paramedic stretcher.

- N.B. Brignoni

Kidney Donor

The nephrologist delivered the news:
your small kidneys,
both functioning
at a terrifying 30 percent.

But everything I have
has your name on it,

even my
organs.

Kidneys or limbs,
you name it,
a sacrifice I'd make
in less than a heartbeat.

- N.B. Brignoni

Love's Words

Words have never fallen from your lips, it's true.
But you're no mute.
In million different ways you speak to my heart you do.

You speak in those smiles,
those sweet hums,
those sparkling eyes that tell me everything.

And oh, how they have become
my favorite sounds
the music of my soul
the catchy song that never leaves
my heart.

A language only love knows.

- N.B. Brignoni

Warrior Pledge

I traded my law school dreams
for a warrior's heart,
standing guard
at your side,

armor and shield in hand.

My heart,
my soul,
always tied to yours.

A choice made,
a sacrifice offered,
late nights and early mornings,
dreams deferred

I'll spend my life
putting you first,
just so I am with you
through every night,
and every day

Any sacrifice
for my universe
is worth any trade.

- N.B. Brignoni

The Only Treatment

No cure, to your rare syndrome

they said.

Just therapy

to manage the symptoms.

So we do

day after day,

hour after endless hour

your tiny body

weary

fighting against itself.

I see it, in the end

of therapy sessions

the struggle in your eyes,

the tremble in your hands

as you fight to learn to crawl.

The sound

of your nose and cheeks

crash into the mat crushes

my heart hurts it tears me up

but then you rise, like you never fell

again and again.

A warrior

in a world of maybes.

This world that doesn't understand

your mighty will

yet.

- N.B. Brignoni

Shark Food

I dream of a cure,
to ease your life.
It's hard to see,
sometimes,
the struggle to stand,
the struggle to crawl,
the struggle of frequent blood draws,
the struggle of seizures,
the struggle to give you daily medicine.

No easy path
for you.

Sometimes this truth
is a shark, chewing away
at my heart.

But we can do this
every day.

I know this is
a life
filled with
triumphs.

And your best chance
at defying
harsh words
is with
therapy's cure
beside your mom
with smiles
and laughs
where you shine.

I'll never leave your side
against the waves of disease
and the carousel of specialists.

We climb
mountains,
always us,
together.

If mountains of pain linger,
then a mountain I'll move for you.

When muscles grow sore,
my arms will always be your getaway,
a trip to home
sweet home.

We rest,
and try again the next day.

- N.B. Brignoni

The fight for a cure, a sum we must all

solve

Have we reached for the stars and planets,
leaving some behind, unwell?

Is a flag on the moon worth more
than a child's peaceful sleep,
untroubled by epilepsy's grip?

Have we lost sight of what truly matters,
the hearts that weep with disease?

We celebrate a moon landing,
a feat of human ingenuity,
but what of the souls in need?
Would it have carried any meaning to them?

Have we truly progressed
if compassion fails to lead?
Are profits placed above healing?

Even S. Jobs, on his deathbed,
knew what truly matters -
connection, love, and legacy.
Why don't we listen?

So I ask once more,
have we truly reached our peak?
When those with cancer, Alzheimer's,
and countless other afflictions
suffer, knowing there isn't a cure within their reach.

Maybe I believe in this new generation more,
as they approach life with open eyes.
Maybe they'll be the ones

to claim the next trophy of human achievement,
to set spirits free from disease.

It would be the first since July 1969.
How many years is that?
Too many.

- N.B. Brignoni

Turn Off Timers to Milestones
Checkmark to your soul's resilience.
Checkmark to your heart's purity.

My little one, these checkmarks
are life's milestones that truly matter.

The ones that will guide you
through any sudden occurrence.

Nothing else on the milestone charts
we see often matters in the end.

- N.B. Brignoni

Girl Full of Sunshine

Sun
in her smile
because it's you
her dad.

Dad at the door— her eyes open wide
with thrill.

She tries to escape the chair
every limb in her body
twists and worms his way.

A yearning to reach her father
though her legs can't move in steps
yet.

But they dream that every person in the room
can see her yearning to run straight
into her father's arms to give him a storm of kisses and
hugs
it's there, even if she can't.

No words escape,
because they can't, yet,
but a glare in her eyes
screams: I love you, Dad.

It's him, the sun in her smile.

A daddy's girl
forever in his warmth
in his sunshine.

- N.B. Brignoni

CHAPTER 4 THE BEAUTY

IN THE BUD'S FORM

The Missing Genes
I must forget the science
because in my eyes
you were made just perfect.

You are my sunflower,
even with missing petals
you bloom always complete to me.

You are my miracle
my universe
whole always complete
to me.

— N.B. Brignoni

Little Warrior Flames

Your light burns
for all to see

it lights a universe
so therefore

You're like the sun
in the daylight

You're like the moon
in the night fall

this place
needs you

you are it's source
of light you belong

Always belonging
to this Earth and it to you

we see you everyday
orbiting our world

making it shine
at every angle

you will always be a star no different
Even with missing
pieces in its form
you still light up
the entire universe

we will always see you

Shine on
little moon

Shine on
little sun

light up this world
near
and far

-N.B. Brignoni

Internet versus Optimism

The internet search bar
a deep dark
sea

A computer
becomes
a place
inside my mind
where my fear is
a violent tide

washing away
the sandcastle
of hope

leaving
questions
about your condition
on cold
sandy feet.

- N.B. Brignoni

The Search

Fingers
tap-tap-tapping
a morse code
of worry
information

floods
drowning my peace
on my
tear-stained face
chest pain
spreads
to stomach
to heart
i should
stop
tapping
but i don't.

- N.B. Brignoni

The Unanswered Questions
the internet a dark sea of what-ifs and
maybes
I search for answers outside of medical
advice I find
videos of families their voices heavy with
grief explaining the disorder with repeating
questions; I hadn't dared to ask flashing
across the screen.
will she read?
will she write?
will she walk down the aisle?
will she hold her own child?
Will she find her soulmate?
the weight of their questions pressing down
on my chest a heaviness that stole my breath
with an ache that could cause a heart to
attack.

So I sought solace outside of videos and explanations.

in online support groups connecting with other parents of children with the same diagnosis. But most of their chats offered no comfort.

I'd asked "how to avoid feeding tubes" I still remember this one mom laughed as she joked about wishing her other child without Wolf-Hirschhorn had a feeding tube it would make it easier for her. While witticism is welcome in this moment, I didn't want to laugh with her I wanted tips and thoughtful suggestions.
I'd been desperate for ways to ease your life to avoid surgeries like a hole in your body a tub to your stomach.

So I searched again for light, for hope, for a glimpse of the sun but found only darkness and more questions the advice every parent seems to have is to grieve the life you imagined.

This crushed my hope for a future of joy rather it planted a seed of doubt fixed in my heart.
So I sought the internet to find a light, stories of joy, a glimpse of the future we could build

but all I found was a black hole of sorrow a
response of questions without answers.

why did it feel so lonely? why couldn't I find
the answers I needed?
You'd think the internet had it all but this
condition was a unicorn.

I noticed that as I scavenged the internet for
positive experiences.

Anyway, I did follow parents their advice as I
grieved the life, I imagined for you a life
where I pictured you as a chess player
beating your father at his own game. Or me
teaching you my favorite sport.

My first love I thought before I met your dad
he stole my heart. But I thought you'd be a
basketball star like your mom. I also pictured
you falling in love with a different sport like
boxing.

Because your dad overprotective said my
daughter will know how to run like a track
star and fight like a professional.

He wanted to make sure you'd always know
to protect yourself. I let this go knowing it's
me I'll be your protector now.

I also mourned the conversations we might
never have as I'd watch children speak to
their parents. It took me a while to not cry at
this sight. Wondering if you and I will ever

get a chance to converse to pick at each
other's brains.

But my grief was utterly paralyzing, advice I
maybe shouldn't have taken too seriously.
Because it took away from your first and
second year of life.

For instance, I regret not reading to you
more, fearing you might not learn. I didn't
want you to feel limited or dependent.

I was too sad to share my day-to-day
activities in the kitchen with you.

Thinking about how maybe you'll never be
able to learn how to cook or bake.

I grieved for the life I thought you'd have this
was an unhealthy process. I didn't do it right
I sank in the grief. And I wasted a lot of time
associating your life with others and crying
every chance.

But I was always looking on the internet for
something more than information and tips, a
path of acceptance and joy.

I wanted to celebrate the unique beauty of
your being.

To find light in the darkness of these seas,
but the internet offered shadows and I was
left feeling more lost and alone in a place
that is supposed to have most if not all the
answers and people a community of support
in one place.

The internet, a vast ocean of information, yet
it couldn't quench my thirst for
understanding. I sought connection, but
found isolation. I yearned for hope, but
stumbled upon despair.

- N.B. Brignoni

Internet stomach pains
i still remember
shaking an eight ball
for answers
if i still had the one back then
i'd trade it in for this laptop's universe
i can't stop typing on with tears
let's face it the internet
is dangerous for a mother
seeking answers unknown
if i had an eight ball
i would've been shaking
for answers
that weren't paralyzing
instead, my fingers shake uncontrollably
in this virtual place with answers
I struggle to accept.
and so

i turned away from the screens
and looked into your eyes
and there, in your silent gaze
i knew i'd have to wait
for you to carve the answers
to the unanswered.
For now, and forever
For in this universe and the next
Loving you always
is the first answer

i'll find.

- N.B. Brignoni

Dearest Past Self

The waves crash, and I know they crash
against your heart too.
We feel things deeply, you and I, and there's
no use pretending otherwise.
I'm reaching back through time, a few years
ahead, offering a glimpse of the sun.
you said you were lost,
searching for
pieces of your heart.
spoiler alert
it was always there,
whole.
it shook,
it beat faster,
but like any muscle,
it grew stronger.
you think you can't swim,
the tide of grief,
overwhelming.

keep swimming.
the water's not in your lungs,
not yet.
Keep swimming. Keep swimming for both of
us.
keep swimming,
towards rainbows,
towards the glimmering horizon.
it gets better.
don't sink.
spoiler alert
she holds a ball
she finds love he's the sun
you'll recognize him when you reach the
shore.
With love and hope,
Your Future Self

- N.B Brignoni

You Glow

a million colors
like a rainbow
everywhere you go
over your head
a colorful arc
so magical
being differently-abled
is your superpower
lucky me
I get to love you
even after
forever

- N.B. Brignoni

white coats drop the ball
they speak of odds
as if bad luck
they number it
one in fifty
thousand
born with
Wolf-Hirschhorn
a ratio I can't
fail to recall

your condition is part of you
but it's the blueprint
of your DNA
and I love every strand

I don't understand
how a genetic specialist
describes a part of you
with a metaphor of a lightning bolt
striking us both

when really you
are the sunrise
after the hurricane
and then some

the rainbow
the unicorn

all the things
lightening
couldn't ever
touch.

- N.B. Brignoni

CHAPTER 5

In this section, we see the beginning of acceptance and adaptation. The poems here deal with coming to terms with the diagnosis, navigating the healthcare system, and more of the early stages of therapy and medical treatment.

Themes include resilience, the search for information and support, and the gradual process of redefining expectations and hopes. These poems also touch on the emotional toll on the family and the process of finding strength in adversity.

This chapter tackles the ongoing medical challenges and emotional turbulence faced by the family. The poems here often use strong rhythms and occasional rhyme to echo the relentless nature of these struggles. Look for ballads that tell the stories of hospital stays and hard-won victories. How will they weather the storms that lie ahead? The strength they've built may be tested in ways they never imagined. But what if the fiercest hurricane is yet to come, one that threatens to uproot everything they've fought so hard to nurture?

Kidney Check up

If they tell us bad news today
my kidney is yours.

If your kidney falls below the marker
below twenty percent my love it is okay

if it is a kidney you must lose
with open arms

I freely give
all of me.

Open me up, open me up
I pray the doctors
let my kidney
take its place.

Let them open me up
no matter the sacrifice.

Let them transplant and mend
you even if it rips me to shreds
whatever it takes.

I'm ready, at any cost
both my hands to the ceiling
you have my heart already
my kidney yours too.

- N.B. Brignoni

Second Birthday Regrets
doctor's
crippling news
lingers in my head
like a bomb
in the middle
of the arcade

kids dance
to a chorus
of happy birthday

two candles
on your cake

but my mind
a year behind
inside the genetics
office

kids scream
becomes tinnitus
the ringing
after my heart's
silent explosion

you on my arm
with a toothy smile

oblivious
to the nuclear
attack inside

happy birthday
they sing
your favorite song

and i tried
i always could

but this time
words wouldn't form

only tears could

the tears
of fear

i gaze at my huge
pregnant belly

your little sister
inside of me
growing
i should've been
strong for her too

but it was the fear
coming back

the one your doctors
instilled in me
it won't leave
that you
may never
ask for the mouse
in character dancing on the dance floor

or scream for cake
like the other kids
in this overcrowded arcade

that truth
a ghost punch
to the gut
it knocked
my mood
down to rock bottom

i'm sorry
i couldn't make it
through the full song
without falling apart

i had to hand you over
to your grandmother

as my eyes rained on your parade
and everyone watched

one of my greatest
regrets

not being strong...

enough, to smile through the entire song

i barely survived

the birthday cake photos

you could tell i was broken
hearted

thanks to fear
always swatting
through the door
without a knock

                    - N.B. Brignoni

Little One
I've made
a million mistakes
these past two years

but none of them
could have ever been
you.

- N.B. Brignoni

the mess in me
grief
the tornado
in my heart
making a mess
round and round
again.

- N.B. Brignoni

when my heart stops bleeding

i shouldn't let my heart
ooze and bleed

but my mind, how it drifts
watching the other kids
and putting
your face in theirs
this is unfair to you
i don't want this

but my mind drifts
uncontrollably
questioning...

if you'll ever feel
what it's like to run
on mulch
and climb
onto the monkey

bars.

Meanwhile, my heart bleeds
from a wound still open.

But soon, the bleeding will stop.
even if it doesn't stop soon,
I'll muster the strength
to play with you,
with the other kids.

i'll be your legs and arms
as i hold you close.

We'll go down every slide
through each ecstatic whirl
it would be just like
you had legs, like other kids
who run carelessly

i'll be your legs forever if i had to
so you too

can run free
and be a kid
with different wings.

- N.B. Brignoni

The Burning Possibilities
I want
to rewrite
our story,
with a future
filled with
possibilities.

But the doctor's bad news
is stuck like a unforgettable record
on replay in the wildfire of my mind
each spot blazing flames
all around.

- N.B. Brignoni

More than Futures

A million futures tucked away
in this soul's book grief sits on a dusty shelf,
reading these words:

I mourn the words unspoken,
the meaningful conversations
we'll never share.

I mourn dance lessons
with your grandma by your side.

I mourn jiu-jitsu teachings
with your father's prideful smile.

I mourn the laughter
we'd share
as we danced badly
together.

I mourn tiny hands that may never
grasp a pen
or bear a wedding ring.

I mourn the books
you may never read.

I mourn you not running
into my arms
when i get home.

I should close this book of grief
every chapter hammering at my soul.

I need to learn to shed
this heavy cloak of mourning.

I shouldn't mourn what could be
because in the end no matter
the page of grief

i'll love you
through it all...

and whatever
comes next
wouldn't
change

a thing.

- N.B. Brignoni

CHAPTER 6 THE STEMS SUSTAIN HURRICANE WINDS

Unfairness' Third Degree Burns

it's no one's fault
when life is unfair to us.
so i've been told everything
happens for a reason.

but i can't
i can't
seem to
make sense of this

new diagnosis: Coxa Valga
a surgery needed
once you turn three.

New Diagnosis: Lazy eye & retina processing issues:
Eye muscle surgery needed
once you turn three.

she's two and i dread the surgical
procedures coming her way

I don't want to picture it

a scalpel cutting through
a body already too fragile.

Wish it were me not you
but Life's unfairness
keeps burning our skin
too often

but then you smile at us
right eyepatch on, tilting your head
and touching the sticker covering your eye -
light again

the sun and the moon, two strong lights combined,
you brought

always pulling a mother and father
out of terror, and back down to earth

so, it's beautiful
even when
it burns.

- N.B. Brignoni

Three Scheduled Surgeries

I hate
that I can't
take your place in the pain
someone should and it should be me.

- N.B. Brignoni

Pinch My Petals Instead

Phlebotomist is taking your blood for the fourth time this
month; you cry and cry until you throw up.

It never gets easier
watching you in pain.
I wish it was me instead.

These thoughts
will never leave me.

take my blood
instead
take my blood
instead.
but they can't
I'm so sorry my baby.

- N.B. Brignoni

Breathing Through the Storm

The feeling hits
when the doctors walk in
with fire and then just start
pouring gasoline.

I know crying in front of my daughter
isn't healthy.

I'm supposed to be stronger
stronger than this.

But why does it have to hurt so much
when they hit me
they hit me every time
with fire and gasoline.

At this stage it feels
like diagnosis after diagnosis,
invasive treatment

after the next invasive treatment,
slowly ripping my heart
into nothing.

I'm still waiting for someone
to just remind me to
inhale & exhale.

But once in a blue moon
it hits me all at once.

Like a wave crashing down
too hard coughing up water
lingering in my lungs.

No wonder I choke
and sometimes
can't form words.

As the doctors wait for responses
on my end approving of surgeries.

But then a tiny sparkle of light:
your small hand
reaching out
to grab my nose
with a smile
and no words

and yet you said
all I needed to hear.

- N.B. Brignoni

Where Rainbows Go

You stopped
the storm
in me

And then, planted
sunflowers
in the aftermath's
debris

You, my brightest
star you remain
always rising

And then, you begin
painting rainbows
on my soul's skin.

- N.B. Brignoni

I Don't Want a Heart of Glass
Your dad
is so strong.

I hate being
the one who cries
in your doctor's office
as they speak of diagnosis, treatments,
and of expectations and medical risks.

I don't want the tissues
or the downpour
of tears...

But they come
anyways.

Why do I

crumble?

I need to be stronger for you, it's true.

I tell myself this in the mirror before appointments,
staring into my own worried eyes: don't break, don't
break.

I say over and over again as if I am preparing for a live
television speech.

But then I break
again
and again
and again.

And then, the next time I look at my reflection
i bite down hard on my teeth and shake my head
in disappointment.

Always feeling like I let you down each breakdown

in the doctor's office is one too many.

- N.B. Brignoni

Doesn't Matter Where We Go

The doctor's thought your path would be a frost-covered slope. One with not many successes only chains of limitations.

But you with a resilient fire in your heart even snow couldn't hold up the tallest snowman our kind has known.

Because you are the sun melting the icy paths they've foresaw.

Doesn't matter where we go. You look beyond the slopes, the storms, and you climb with the sun.

I love how you move in your own unicorn ways.

- N.B. Brignoni

Mom's Shattered Armor

It doesn't feel real
your eyes vacant, lost
searching the ceiling
six minutes into the seizing.

A sound like glass breaking
my motherly armor is shattering.

I once thought my motherly armor could shield you

from anything.

But oh, how i hate science
a cold goddess for not always
letting me keep you safe.

Because it is still so surreal
your vacant eyes
stare back beside me

I lie there with you
waiting for the moment
you come back waiting for your body
to stop the scary convulsions.

It doesn't feel real.

It never feels real
you are only two.

- N.B. Brignoni

The Weight of the Earthquakes

your voice, trapped behind the seizure

neurons that misfire and muscles that betray

i scream in a silence so loud

it deafens me while the 911 dispatcher calls to me

I would give my own voice

to hear just one word from yours

what i would give to stop the tremors on your body

i'd give up everything

to take away your seizures

in your sleep, so you can dream.

- n.b. brignoni

CHAPTER 7 MOONLIT PETALS STARGAZING

Nightmares Where I Saw Sunflowers

Another nightmare of a plane crash on the
highway.

This time I wasn't afraid to run towards the
cockpit of the of jet.

Fearful, as I was, I told myself if my kids
were on that plane i'd want a good
Samaritan to try and save them.

But the plane was empty no passengers only
a Sunzilla sunflower missing petals.

But where petals should be there was flames.

This sunflower had eyes like yours. And I
thought to myself it's you isn't it you are
shining your light in my nightmares.

I knew I was asleep, watching the sunflower
arching high, staring at me so I pinched
myself awake.

My eyes opened, realizing even in a bad
dream

you came shining your light, forcing me to
wake.

You came, little sunflower and you saved me
so cleverly from my common airplane
nightmare.

Even nightmares aren't the same now that
you exist.

Even in bad dreams i've become stronger
because of you i've become less afraid.

- N.B. Brignoni

The Crown of Wires She Wears
You wear science
on your head
and I smile.

Because any fabric
placed on your skin
is picture-perfect.

Science is testing
your brainwaves
for seizure activity.

Meanwhile i admire the tiny
sensors, circling your head
with a hair net it is like wired-perfection.

You make science
look so beautiful baby.

- N.B. Brignoni

The EEG Crown Of Gentle Observers

Your brain, a beautiful city with a billion
neurons.

Neurons that are beeping, flashing, guiding,
buzzing alive like a mardi gra parade in New
Orleans.

But when a seizure strikes it's as if a meteor
shower, is disrupting the flow of your brain's
bright city.

A billion neurons lights are extinguished,
and darkness falls like turning off the lights
in a basement.

For your brain still growing in size the
power lines severed, and the neurologicl
streets plunged into chaos, a brain blackout.

When seizures stop and lights in the city
turn back on it just leaves a mark in
lightning's trace on my heart.

Each spike, each wave, the sensors catch
during testing brings me to ground on my
knees praying we can make it through
blackouts togther each time. And a
realization of a diagnosis, I am not ready to
hear.

- N.B. Brignoni

No Wooden Nose
they ask, "are you okay?"
i nod yes with a smile at your beautifully
unaware expression
thankfully
i am no Pinocchio,
you don't understand epilepsy

but the news wraps
around my neck like a rope
being pulled over and over again
no cure they said
only a trial-and-error process
of medicine rituals
my mind spiraling in panic,
terrified of the next seizure

but you, my strong one
i will smile for you

i will find the strength
you need me to show

i smile for now. Even though inside i am
crumbling, curled in a fetal position, crying

because I can't protect you from this
I'm not okay

thankfully
no wooden nose
to grow and betray the words
i cough out
watching you laugh adorably
while my smile a mask hiding
my breaking heart

but for you my love
i'll be strong
even when strength
feels like a stranger to me

for you i will be strong even when
i am not strong for me a lesson i never
learned

but for you i am strong
always for you a lesson not taught
it felt more like second nature.

N.B. Brignoni

Neurology Results

EEG found
brain spikes

only in restful states

i never saw
sleep the same
paranoid you'll be seizing
while I sleep

not even
in my dreams
do i want to drift too far
far from where you sleep

not when there is no cure
for epilepsy.

- N.B. Brignoni

The Unwanted Stamp

Your neurologist
formally diagnoses you with "Focal Epilepsy"

I was not ready for this truth,
another illness to stamp on records.

We dreamt of a world
where you could run free
of worries.

But reality gave you
a different path
one where you
have to fight
for every step
you take.

- N.B. Brignoni

The Weight We Carry

mama's armor
a fragile facade
concealing a heart of glass

a heart
always seemingly to be
on the brink of shattering.

the ticking bomb of tears
tick a constant threat to my soul.

while in the sofa's shadow, I hide
in the dark corners of my mind.

the television's glow
a distraction for you

as I view new neurology
test results that are too bitter
to swallow

reminding me of another
battle we must
fight together

each diagnosis
another stone
weighing heavy
on your tiny
shoulders

this isn't like a kidney
but if it was i'd volunteer
to give you my brain

i'd take yours
so i can take
the forever
diagnosis
of epilepsy and free you
from its chains.

but my heart breaks
in a million different ways
knowing i can't save or stop
the seizures that have yet to come.

epilepsy a diagnosis
a heavier stone
like a yellow bus
on your shoulders

i wish I could lift each stone you hold
on Hypotonia bones but some burdens
can't be shared even by a willing parent

so, I turn back to the sofa's corner.

i cry

i break

hidden from your innocent eyes yet, even as
tears fall like rain.

and my heart's fragile state is exposed

i will stand beside you, through seizures
through anything frightening like a mama
bear shielding her cub.

And with the strength and superpower of the
woman with the S on her chest.

Maybe I'm starting to get
my supermom cape back.

- N.B. Brignoni

The Dangerous Dances in Your Dreams

The results from the EEG finally arrived,
explaining your frequent seizures.
I read them over and over again in disbelief.
Heartbroken by your neurologist's findings.

But your smile is infectious in the
background.
I had to stop reading the results on my
phone.
To kiss your cheeks again and again.
They were goodnight kisses
filled with fear as your bedtime is here.

My mind replays mornings when I wake up
and your eyes are vacant
an absent seizure took your body.

And I wish I knew when it all started.

Now, I live in constant fear.
When I wake, will you not be here?

Or will you be gone, my voice unheard to
your ears
you in a place I can't reach, even when you
are right next to me.

Moments like this, I wish epilepsy didn't
exist.

- N.B. Brignoni

Sticks, Stones, and Sunflowers

Holes in my heart, the world
throws sticks and stones
at my window.

Yet I still open the curtains
to the light because I want to
bloom beside you.

- N.B. Brignoni

Every time You Rest

A noiseless battle fought
with every shutting
of your brown eyes
as they drift off to sleep.

And when you drift off
I can't help but watch you
sleep worried while you dream
I never see sleep.

- N.B. Brignoni

Sky Falls
Even when the sky cracked open
a million stars
raining down on you

A small fighter
with a big light
in a unfair World

But you a blazing sun
a supernova against the darkness
your little body fighting
battles bigger than most

But your light
never dims
even when
the sky shatters
and your body
becomes an earthquake
know that even if your eyes
roll backwards, even if the sky falls
before us i will be the light you need
to bring you back and hold up the sky
at the same time.

I hope you
know when your eyes
roll back and your body seizes.

I am here with you always

my hands outstretched

as the sky falls
i catch the pieces
and begin piecing it
back together

holding you up to light
to help you find your way
out of your brains blackout.

Together we are unbreakable
against the seizures.

                    - N.B. Brignoni

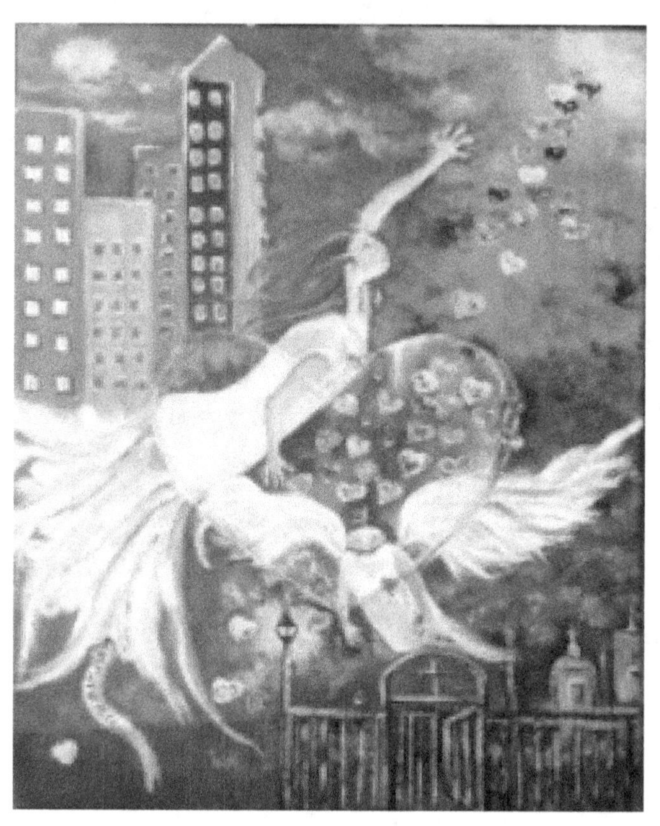

CHAPTER 8 STARLIGHT PETALS

We Hear a Love Unspoken

On Father's Day, it will sting to see
daughters share stories kept.

You yearn to hear hers
we have both wished for it.

Our daughter is different
from the others.

More like the trees & clouds
no words, only sweet hums of the rustling
leaves and cotton colors
telling stories the wind carries.

Our daughter silently strong
because her heart speaks
when you're near, all can tell
she's in awe of you

Like a sunflower turning to the sun
she does the same always towards you

Not me

No words needed
her eyes confess daddy's girl
always and forever you are her sun in the
flesh.

- N.B. Brignoni

Crowded Rooms

the world assaults
you a sensory storm
i want to make disappear for you
lights too bright, sounds too loud

workers begin stocking the shelfs
tall like a mountain.

the objects stack quicker and quicker
and the workers move faster and faster

you get upset it's too much
movement and begin turning your body
ready to jump out my arms.

i watch you retreat into your shell
of fear and anxiety

i begin wishing i could build a bubble
to keep out the chaos that short-circuits
your senses

i want to wash away the pain
you feel

but i can't so i hurts me too when you and i
are in a crowded room i wish i knew how i
could help you...

-n.b. brignoni

Medical Odds Don't Share Ears

Your doctor had said
you might not ever talk,
nonverbal, you may stay.

But she doesn't hear with my ears:
you speak to my heart
all the time, in many forms.

The tune you sing never stops
it is my heart and soul's favorite song.

- N.B. Brignoni

Hearts Awake

You are the kind of sun
that melts the snow
my special daughter
forever grow in your
out of the ordinary
ways.

- N.B. Brignoni

You're My Peace Love

I love
holding you

as you fall asleep.

It's the place
where I let my
anger just goes like an exhale.

- N.B. Brignoni

Five days of therapy
Five days of therapy
each day I am honored
to witness your strength.

It's contagious,you inspire me every day
to write these words on this page.

Because of you I am able
to share your resilient story—
one you've written for me, clearly
one full of miracles and trials.

Trials, you seem to battle
like a well-trained warrior.

I couldn't be any prouder
to pick you up from each therapy session
 through every win and struggle
we celebrate
with high-fives
and ice cream smiles.

- N.B. Brignoni

Always Love's Open Arms

Even if your feet don't walk one in front of the other.

Even if your voice stays in hums and not words.

To me, you'll always be like a sunflower blooming golden
and bright in my garden, perfect as you stand.

You don't have to change for me i'll love you in every form.

- N.B. Brignoni

The Heart Bleed
Mama's heart-attacking
while her daughter's
tiny body trembles
as neurons spike,
in her brain.

"No, not again!" she yells.

She is begging the universe
to give her daughter's body
a break.

Her knees were still blue
from all the praying
every night.

A silent sky doesn't speak, but the seizure
stops.

A mother's cuts bloom into scars on her
heart.

But one more cut still bleeds.

- N.B. Brignoni

Purple Knees and Prayers

She shouldn't have to fight multiple
disorders at once.

A little girl deserves to dream at night, not
have a tonic seizure in her sleep.

And all I could do was pray at one in the
morning.

I slamed my knees on to the holy ground

And I prayed about one hundred times on
purple knees till her eyes came back to life.

The seizure passes, and the sound of sirens
gets closer.

Her life could never be routine
as her brain spikes when she sleeps.

Where and when can my little girl find
peace?

This kind of cruel science will never make
any sense to me.

-N.B. Brignoni

CHAPTER 9

The Oceans Weight

You shouldn't carry burdens meant for the sea.

Your strength shouldn't have to carry burdens that deep.

Tiny hands shouldn't hold such heavy things.It's cruel at your age to spend more time in hospitals and not zoos.

Tiny hands were meant for toys. Not for needles that are sharp, pierce, and burn.

I see you, my moon, with tired bone after the seizure caused its quake shaking every part of your tiny form.

And now you rest, eyes closed on the hospital bed too big for your frame.

Though, even here you are tiniest but still i see your strength as you sleep peacefully.

You are so strong, the strongest in the room.

- N.B. Brignoni

storms & rainbows
sometimes when your doctor talks
and you find my eyes

you'll see i am a storm
no dam could hold.

i'm still learning how to deal with fear and not
fall apart in front you.

sometimes in the doctors office i am the driving
rain but together will make a rainbow.

- n.b brignoni

FaceTime with Her Dad

First words not spoken

yet but every movement

in her body speaks.

As she moves away

from the nurse a trick to escape

the draw of blood but needles prick.

A mother holds her hand

but she cries the blood draw too much pain

But then it's him

on the phone her sun

all he does is talk

and she listens.

She speaks in her silence

every word felt, as her breathing slows

with her dad on the screen.

and in her silence, eyes stare into his

he understands her language and responds.

Even far away

his love reaches like hands

that hold hers he is

a shield against pain

daddy's girl

always.

- N.B. Brignoni

You Speak in Dreams

you are non-verbal
but in my dreams
you are a river of words
flowing freely

last night, i spoke first
and then woke up in tears

i play the dream back like a memory
it is you holding my hand
you speak sweet things in sentences

a tease that breaks me
leaving me to wonder

what games this universe plays
does it conspire
to bring us together
in the night?

since i never want to sleep
when you do

maybe someone knew
we needed more than
reality

we also needed to find each other even in dreams
your full sentence replays in my ears
on repeat.

- n.b. brignoni

my unicorn butterfly
i believed in you
before the developmental delays
led us to the maybe
you won't walk or talk.

and still, i believe in you now
as i believe every caterpillar
can metamorphosize.

you'll get your butterfly wings,
rainbow-like
and strong.

they will be wings of a different kind
and with them, you'll find a way to fly.

my unicorn butterfly
this giant ecosphere
yours to explore

- N.B. Brignoni

Bedtime Peace
Next to me you
breathe, and I sleep
so peacefully.

- N.B. Brignoni

Flower in Class

I am a flower, still learning not to bend

and not break in a hurricane's presence.

-N.B. Brignoni

Tainted Metaphors

I didn't like your geneticist's metaphor
for your condition because you are more like a winning
lottery ticket.

But they'll say, it's like a lightning strike
with a tsunami of maybes.

So, my little warrior you must know the most imporant
truth.

You are not a genetic tragedy.

You are not defined by odds or maybes.

Rather, you are a galaxy forming, a universe expanding.
You are a big bang theory of your own.

A hold a universe of strength that lightning couldn't touch.

- N.B. Brignoni

He's Her World

a knocking on the
hospital door

he open's it's you, her father
he's her world in human form.

- N.B. Brignoni

warrior's heart and soul
tiny hands
hold a universe
of strength

even with big burdens
on her back the weight of every sea clings on
to her but she keeps going.

if resilience could be a person it would be
you, my little warrior you never fall without
getting back up

- N.B. Brignoni

CHAPTER 10

The Box We Haven't Escaped

Ambulance sirens straight to you again a cycle that repeats. It's not the sounds I craved for your young ears to hear so often as you do.

I had a yearning for you to hear the sounds of swings creaking, slides squealing, and the kids' laughter echoing from the monkey bars.

But your hand barely bigger than my thumb warms mine on the hospital bed.

I was about to let go. I had thought you'd been fast asleep (postictal seizure state) but your fighter's grip tightened around one of my fingers.

Your eyes open slowly.
I smile then you smile.

The machines continue
their relentless beeping
a rhythm both familiar and terrifying.

These four white walls
became a box
we haven't been able
to escape from just yet.

I'm sorry my love.

The children's hospital
isn't the second home
i dreamt of for us
but soon this box
will leave.

I begin to say, "I'll buy us ice cream afterwards.
I'll take you to the playground down the street. I think you
are ready to play with the big kids."

I lift my head off the bed to see your response, but you went
back to sleeping.

And I became lost in the hum of machines.
The ambulance wail still replaying in my aching heart.

- N.B. Brignoni

We Dreamt of Oceans

With sandcastles not of hospital beds
and doctor rotations.

But little one, this will just be the part of our story
that builds our resilience

- N.B. Brignoni

Rainbow walls

Hospital walls
a canvas
for our love

143

to paint rainbows
over the dark

together
we paint hope
on blank walls
and over fear's darkness

an art piece worthy of a museum
tiny hands guided by
mother's love

brushstrokes of a future outside
of this box

a place bathed in sun these walls witness
our masterpiece of resilience and love.

- N.B. Brignoni

CHAPTER 11

The Fire On Neptune

A little spark, your flame flies
against the doctors' frozen forecasts years
back.

Yet you do not freeze—
you're a supernova without an explosion.

While white coats charted a course
through Neptune's giant storms,
a path less traveled, an icy unknown,

You glided through the ice,
with a heart the size of Jupiter,
never letting it chill your bones.

Like a comet's tail, you blaze
through the icy paths
where no fire existed once before.

You a star that spits fire in the wind of resilience;
inside the ice giant, you didn't freeze.

Your strength is blooming still,
in the fire, the spark in your soul,
a tank fueled by mighty desire and love.

You learn as you fall and rise,
it is you who reinvented the unknown

and created a garden of your own.

On Neptune, never forget you are a sun
melting the ice giant's heart thawing what
was once cold.

I never doubted your powers.

Not once.

Keep growing strong you will always be loved.

- N.B. Brignoni

hope lives in therapies glow

therapy's garden
you are loved
a sunflower
always tended

your therapist's heart
blooms for you
like a child of their own
that's when i knew i had chosen
the perfect place for you

therapist with the sun
on their side
guide your tiny hands to reach
bubbles
but your tiny legs fall
they catch you midway

five days a week
a mountain we climb
in sync
we won't stray
each milestone met
a new seed planted
of possibilities

therapy's glow
a sunflower
spitting fire
in the frost of
maybe she will not
your strength
shows burning their doubts

in therapy's embrace
every success and fall counts
"cannot do"
is banished
every flower finds their way
guided by courage and light

in therapy's place
a garden of beautiful wildflowers
reaching for sun

but you easy to spot a sunflower who stands out with the
flames of resilence at her core. And more fire where petals
fell.

i see the beauty in everything, even fallen petals that led to
the fires that light up my world

i don't care what any profesional says you are and always
have been born my perfect sunflower.

- n.b. brignoni

the magic you made with lemons

i see your limbs
reaching for colorful blocks
smooth and cool

small legs
wobbly, tiny hands
fumbling a block far away

but determined
to learn those first steps, reaching far
though your legs don't
stand yet

they try
legs shaky
you fall
with a puff of air
that could blow
a piggie's house
down

but you get back up
with a silly smile, tongue sticking out
and stand a few seconds more

the therapist guides
your legs, encourages another step
even if you stumble
my pride bursts

life gave you lemons, and you squeeze
every bit with magic.

-n.b. brignoni

i won't stop believing in you
i recall another night
in my dreams last night
where you speak to me.

I stay silent in disbelief
till I wake

and wonder why
I've heard you speak
in my dreams more than once

sometimes it hurts

to dream

knowing

what might

never be real.

but I still do
believe in you

even if it stings
my silent hope
has never left

one day you and i will
talk about our day
in words and sentences.

-n.b. brignoni

Wolf-hirschhorn Warrior

missing genes
can't ever dim
the star
that you are
my love
nothing
can

-n.b. brignoni

The Genetic Deletion

Genetics deleted
on chromosome four
it may carve a path
only two percent
have walked
through
before

it may very well
cause a delay in
speech and motor skills

but things if you do

meet milestones or don't

either way you are a star

that will shine at every angle

without question

-n.b. brignoni

the perfect dad, yours

maybe his daughter
won't take first steps
yet in his arms
she'll fly
always

-n.b. brignoni

No Fear

As your little

knees buckle and your body falls forward

your face falls first onto the soft, blue

gymnastics mat an attempt to stand.

I watch you, watch
another kid dart by, so fast
the mat beneath you shakes
so hard it rocked you
out of your sitting position.

it hurts to watch
and not be able
to catch you when you
fall

in therapy sessions
it's a lesson to fall
a lesson you know well

but you know what
you seem to always
get back up with a smile

as i watch you determined, your tongue out
taking a few breaths and you try to stand
again

a few seconds more on your feet,
and you smile, proud.

it's that smile,
the fire in your eyes, to not give up

my strong girl
always leaving me
awe-struck

-n.b. brignoni

there is magic in missing petals

there is magic in missing petals
you are living proof

miracles bloom
even in
the dry

dessert soil

even
with
missing
petals

little one you bloom
differently than others
but it gives you a shine of your own

i am no longer afraid
of the future by the way you shine

i should've know better
this world is yours to write
it never was the doctor's place

now i know you were
born with a resilience and special shine only
will illuminate the path of fallen petals
for others to follow

because there is magic in missing petals
on chromosome four

and you
are the
living proof

- n.b. brignoni

miracles don't have to wait

i don't have to

wait for a miracle

anymore because my little one

every day

i get to gaze at you

i see

it's you,

my miracle

come true

Gait Trainer Evaluation

New specialist
only read
the diagnosis
under your name.

When she mumbles
under her breath
she doubts your strength.

She says no
to wheels that move
to help you learn steps.

But you stay still
as she waves obnoxiously
to come her way or mine.

I explain bubbles are your favorite
thing to see like a toy.

And I explain it could be used as motivation
for you to move.

I request the therapist to get the bubbles she
has in the next room for you to have fun.

She scoffs and mutters under her breath
doubting it'll make a difference
but goes to grab them anyways.

She begins blowing bubbles
and your statue crumbles

as you reach, legs move with wheels
you take steps toward the bubbles

your first steps
on video i knew you could
i never doubt you

my heart explodes
the specialist nods
"okay, i think she's ready."

a gait-trainer referral at last
you did it and she didn't believe
bubbles would make a difference

but i know your language

you can always count on me to be your
words
and sentences.

-n.b. brignoni

Never Silent Again I Roar For you

I never

understood

the power

of my voice

until it became

yours

too

-N.B. Brignoni

The Little Girl on the Moon

Watching you
take your first steps
on the gait trainer.

Was just like watching
the astronauts on July 21, 1969
put a flag on the moon.

- N.B. Brignoni

CHAPTER 12

morning rituals

every day you wake
without a seizure

i kiss your forehead
good morning

and thank
my lucky stars

while i dispense
your daily medicines

an exhale out
i am relieved of the medicines magic.

-n.b. brignoni

Seizures on Streets

first steps
with gait trainer
a celebration
cut short

you fell asleep
on the drive home

bones tired from
taking steps

then suddenly
you woke up
vomitting
all over
your carseat

i pull over
and then, you begin
to have seizure
as i take you
out the carseat

you were an
earthquake
in my arms

i placed
you on the van's
trunk lied you down
onto your side.

I try to remember
the name of the road

I feel I failed you
not knowing

what road, we were on
when the 911 dispatcher asked
my mind a blank, my eyes only on you
afraid this seizure felt scarier

your body convulsing
vomit across the van's interior
counting the slow stirring time

i had been ready this time
with emergency medicine
to attempt to stop the seizure

now seizures on streets
a new parental fear to overcome

i didn't know the road

instead all I knew
when four minutes passed
and you were still in your seizure
state.

i had doctor's orders to give
you the medicine to stop your
body's quake.

i couldn't be more,

thankful for the cop
who saw us and
saw you in the back
of the van floor trembling

he called for help

he knew the road

and four minutes

just passed

it was time
to give you
the medicine
i begin to prepare it

but then you wake
as I was about to administer it
with a sideways smile on your face

my little sun
always shining bright
always so strong
you don't seem to fear much
you don't bend and break
you bend and become stronger

as you smile
coming out of this seizure on the side
of a busy road.

-n.b. brignoni

Sirens Straight to You

As the paramedics
place you, on the stretcher.

I wanted to tell you your epilepsy
wouldn't last forever.

I couldn't form the words.

As I hold my hand
to my nose and mouth

My chest pains began worsen
as i try to muffle back the tears knowing i
couldn't lie to you epilepsy was forever.

But i won't say that out loud
it hurts too much to say so.
- N.B. Brignoni

hospital shower breaks hide salty trails

your toddler body
a combat zone
facing struggles too soon

my soul is sad
this life of constant battles
i wouldn't wish for any child
especially my own

my soul, a dam
it carries tears of rivers
ready to pour but i hold

as i go to the shower
a ritual of escape

heartbroken
my body is weak

mind in the dark
my tears fall

like rain in a thunderstorm

all masked
in showers downpour

shower water
hides salty trails

it hides
the breaking of me
from everyone else

-n.b. brignoni

a wish to bring you the ocean
you can't sleep
without the sounds of the waves
crashing

but tonight
after the seizure
left your body

i daydreamed
we were there
as i listened to the ocean
sounds and watched you rest

muting out
the beeping
of hospital
machines

as i gazed at you sleeping while my mind
drifts, dreaming of us, we were happy
building sandcastles

i had you in my arms
leaving the sandcastles behind us
and then we searched the sand for seashells

we found one
as big as my cellphone

but then the doctor walks in
the dream dissolves
with more news of more medicines
to try, to stop seizures
in your sleep

now, every time
we find ourselves
back in this hospital bed

i wish i could toss the ocean
at your feet so we can play in the sand
walk the ocean embrace the beauty of nature

because this hospital
is no place for children
to always be

but i bring you the ocean
in my dreams.

- n.b. brignoni

Sweet Dreams

of all the dreams

i love to dream

about you the most

- n.b. brignoni

You Talk in My Dreams

You are non-verbal.
It wasn't real, but it always feels real.

It's as if we both go to sleep together
and meet again in dreams.

This dream was different from others.

This time I spoke first.

And I woke with a smile instead of tears.

I recall this dream like a memory once again.

My dreams becoming easier to remember
as i think back to this one.

"The moon," I said, "it stares at me."

Confused, Athena, "Where?" she'd ask. My finger, hesitant,
pointed at her face. A silly giggle escaped me.

"No, silly goose," she lifts her tiny hand out of the hospital
sheets and points out the window at the full moon.

"No look, it's right there!"
I insisted with giggles, pointing again at her.

This time she screams, "Mom, I am not the moon! Look, it's
right there!"

Her voice then cracked, a laugh that rose as I grabbed her
close.

"No, look at you! You are my moon. So strong, always
finding ways to glow. You are like a lamp in a dark
room." My words spoke slow.

Athena tilts her head, eyes confused again.

She says, "No, I am not a lamp or a moon, are you
okay? Should I call the doctor?" She starts belly
laughing till she cries.

Both of us lost in laughter on the hospital bed
that started feeling like home.

The dream begins to fade,
I hug you tighter until it was gone.

I run to your bed as you wake
and say, "You are my moon."
And you smile almost about to giggle like you knew.

Maybe you and I
we talk in dreams together, another

unicorn way of yours.

-N.B. Brignoni

not meant to be

dark skies keep coming back
a wish blue skies

but another seizure
in your sleep and the lightening strikes me

another night i
wake up to your eyes
vacant your body an earthquake

dark skies keep hovering us
i keep making wishes for blue skies

but wishes don't shift the storm
in your small body

I used to believe in reasons
for everything but can't make one for this

my little girl is too young for such lessons
my heart disappears, searching for its
meaning

but nothing is ever meant
just a coin flip in the air heads or tails isn't?

- n.b. brignoni

the light I lose when she seizes

here she is, my sun
but no sunlight
kisses my face

and no warmth
is felt in my bones

the sky is ice-cold
when the seizure
strikes her soul

and then steals her dreams
for minutes
too long

-n.b brignoni

cradled in my arms will go

tiny legs
not walking
yet

but there is no rush
my little one

to a finish line

cradled
in my arms
you'll go

wherever
your heart
desires

curtains open
a world
of your making

my legs
are yours

my arms
your ship
we'll sail every sea

kiss
every shore
cradled in my arms

i will be your ship
always at your service
wherever your heart desires

-n.b. brignoni

gravity is heavy

all six of my shoulder's bones
begin to break
under the weight

of her epilepsy

a building
of past seizures
stacked tall
have built
a building that could
touch the sky

but i want to find a way
to break it down

to save her from the gravity
of it all

but it is heavy, the stones piled high
and seizures
keep coming
without pause
stones fall

i wonder
if you can hear me now
Sky?

as i dry her tears
they pour down
my shirt soaked

leaving the hospital
she's tired, fighting sleep
after a long night

and now the sun sets
again, and my head bows

how do we make sense
of something of this magnitude

Sky?

seizures they keep shaving time
off her dreams and precious sleep.

Sky you can't stop them give her peace?

i beg, i pray, to the sky a million times on my blue knees.

but here we are, leaving the
hospital again for the fifth time
this month.

- n.b. brignoni

seashells and sunflower wishes

what is the reason?
if everything has a purpose,
this one doesn't make sense.

my little one
is an ocean lover
who's never been to the beach

she lays, on the hospital bed
and i wish it were me instead.

i'd take the pain of piercing needles,
iv's and blood draws,
take the seizures.
take it all.

so you could go explore
another place, outside of here.

a place to adventure
to find seashells on the beach
like a toddler would.

i want to pull you from this bed, take you to the beach play in
the sand, smell the salt in the air, feel the sun kiss your face.

we'd leave handprints in the sand, build sandcastles together.
But then the tide comes strong you and scream and laugh as
we watch the waves crashing, breaking the castles we built in
half.

but reality is nothing like my daydreams.

my heart breaks in two, trying to make sense of every
hospital visit.

for now, i let go of making sense of the situation
embracing you skin to skin giving you kisseson this hospital
bed is the only answer that makes sense.

the waves will wait for us

and when we make it to the beach we will make up for lost
time in hospital rooms

- n.b. brignoni

CHAPTER 13

you redefine perfect genes

in a world
of perfect dna

i'd still want yours
with its missing pieces

white coats count, but all they see
is your genetic deletion, as they say 54 genes
gone astray

but i see
a mosaic of you

you are whole
in every imperfect

you are more
than they can see

to me
you'll always
be complete

not missing a thing

- n.b. brignoni

beachside remedy

One day soon my face will wear less worry.

When your seizures, i pray, take a rest.

I'll carry you, unafraid of blue lips, and take
you not to the usual therapy or doctors
appointments.

But to the bridge connected to the beach,
straight to the sand and salty air.

Our bottoms planted on the shore's edge.
Our toes feeling the cold waves crash.
Our hands sandy, sticky with melting ice
cream. One of mine holding you up steady,
the other grips a cone.

Our faces kissed by the sunshine, while you
wear a picture-perfect vanilla ice-cream
smile.

This plan of ours, a small taste of being two,
a universe away from beeping machines, just
us, making up for time missed.

- n.b. brignoni

heartsick sounds

Sirens roar a trigger—
anxiety floods my chest
tingling sensations
like electricity

my heart plummets

to my stomach
heartsick

no medicine
for this paranoia

even if they aren't coming
toward the house

my brain
still thinks they are

another conversation
to be held with my therapist.

- n.b. brignoni

Birthday Betterments

First birthday
the seizure's ghost
lingering like a heavy dark cloud
over my head my smile broken.

Second one
tears stopping the fire
on your birthday cake.

Third birthday has yet to come
but this one i can promise to be the sun
you always deserved.

- n.b. brignoni

Mountains Trophies

You, the miracle
that guided my growth,

I couldn't have found the strength
to climb mountains as tall as the Rockies
without your love and resilence.

Your strength and spirit have nurtured my own.

I wouldn't have evolved this much without you.

- n.b. brignoni

how could i go?
i never
want to go
when i look at you
my heart it is so full

- n.b. brignoni

CHAPTER 14 THE BLOOMING OF THE WILDFLOWERS

The Story of a Warrior Sunflower
Missing petals, yet blooming still
strength found in every challenge
and every step forward

I pen the progress
because you will always be
the greatest story I have to tell.

-N.B. Brignoni

The Ode of Being Undeniably You

disabled
you are not

you shine
while wheels spin

a million colors
bursting forth

a personal rainbow
following you

beautifully different
perfect as is.

maybe they say
disabled

but no labels
will ever stick

lucky though
every sunrise
a world is painted with rainbows

all thanks to you glistening
like diamonds do

always in therapy
with the diamond sparklings light

How could we all not be
awestruck head over heals enraptured, and utterly in love
with you as you are?

-N.B. Brignoni

Strongest Legs

Oh, I'm obsessed with how you move those tiny yet strongest legs. I know you don't walk like the other kids in the therapy room.

But I love your walk more. It comes with the sounds of metal wheels clanky towards me, slow serenades.

I know you're still learning; your legs buckle and go back up.

One foot in front of the other with the sounds of metal wheels clanky towards me, slow serenades.

Every wobble down I see the strength it takes to rise but you do it with a trophy smile.

I know the doctors said this moment might not come.

But your trembling legs take you places the metal wheels clanking towards me, slow serenades.

It's a walk of defiance.
Every inch forward is a miracle.

Look at you go my unicorn!
My hand is on my chest—I'm so obsessed!

My eyes full of tears.

-N.B. Brignoni

Unicorn Steps

Another day, another therapy
victory lap filled with wheels
moving & steps though legs fall
but flappy muscles & all
you rise again

You carry
Hercules strength
with Athena's spirit

I, the proud mama camera ready
to capture the evidence of your resilience.

-N.B. Brignoni

Haiku Hearts of Courage Found Here

From tears, rainbows bloom
stories weave threads of courage
brave hearts, we rise up.

- N.B. Brignoni

Doctor's Crystal Ball Broken?

They wrote your future in dark shades of blue.
Handed me blueprints of limitations a scary pamphlet full
of gloom.

A first-time mother broken scanning the list with tsunami
of tears hidden in shadows.

Your dad didn't let you see me as I empty the tissue box.
But white coats couldn't see the rainbow's arc
shimmering above your head a billion colors bright.

Your future even then a mixture of light and magic.
The sun shining through every therapy struggle.

Every medical battle fought.
I had to forget the milestone boxes unchecked.

And remember only your genetic code
makes you a beautiful anomaly

forever rare
and mine to cherish
endlessly.

- N.B. Brignoni

lost time defusing the bomb

doctors' news
use to be the grenade
jumping in my heart
waiting to blow

ticking
ticking
ticking

until i let go of all they said
she might not do

so the grenade's
ticking
ticking
ticking
like a clock of fear
stopped

the grenade clucking in my heart
is gone
when i saw you
perfect as is

- n.b. brignoni

The Navigation System Never Broken

No matter
where we go

No GPS is necessary
with a love as nourishing as yours

I could never
forget my way home.

- N.B. Brignoni

Love you Dearly
You are the place
where I find my peace.

And you don't
even know it.

Oh my sweet baby
you don't have to
change a thing.

You make me so happy.

-n.b. brignoni

CHAPTER 14 FLOWERS

WHOLE

Flourishing New Petals

Being a mom again, noticing day by day
it isn't like the first time.

I see it now.

What the doctors once saw in my first-born.

But she will always be my normal.

Or maybe nothing is meant to be normal.

Maybe every parent should see their children
like it is their first time.
And not hold them to standards of "normal" rather just
create a life where normal isn't something we seek rather
something we hear of as we all create our normal in our
own unique style.

- n.b. brignoni

Mom for the Second Time

I felt the whole world
slow down when your sister was born

I was waiting for another shoe to drop
for this pregnancy to be scarier
than the last time.

But your sister much like you is warrior too
she made it to this world without an illness to find.

-n.b brignoni

It's warmer with two.

One daughter
on each arm
smiling and laughing.

Not enough
lifetimes to hold you
two like this.

This moment I take a picture in my mind
and think to myself that I couldn't have
dreamt of something
this perfect.

- N.B. Brignoni

Mother's Day

They ask
for a gift ideas
for a perfect mother's day gift.

As I watch them
my daughters
the light in their eyes
laughing with their father

And then
a click like a
a lightbulb switch

Answering their questions
no need for a box
with ribbons and bows

My heart is whole
two perfect gifts
already mine their
priceless

- N.B. Brignoni

My Daughters
are heaven sent
the way they
always
lift me up
from my mind's
rock bottom
without a touch
just a smile
or a laugh like magic, I rise
stronger than i've ever been because of them.

-n.b brignoni

Sirens With a New String to Pull

Six months old blissfully
unaware of the seizure
that shook her sister's world.

She smiles at the stretcher's wheels
that carries her sister.

An ache in my chest.
One day I'll have to find the words
to teach you of the seizures and sirens.

But most of all strength.

You'll soon see it's engraved
in your name Aesira (stands for)—Fearless

So when the sirens hush and all is still.

You'll soon see it's in your sister's name too

Athena—Warrior.

- N.B. Brignoni

195

Home Has No Snooze Buttons

You make me appreciate
the little things in life
even more.
You made me
realize time
time is
as precious
as you

-N.B. Brignoni

Two Roads Lead to Love's Home

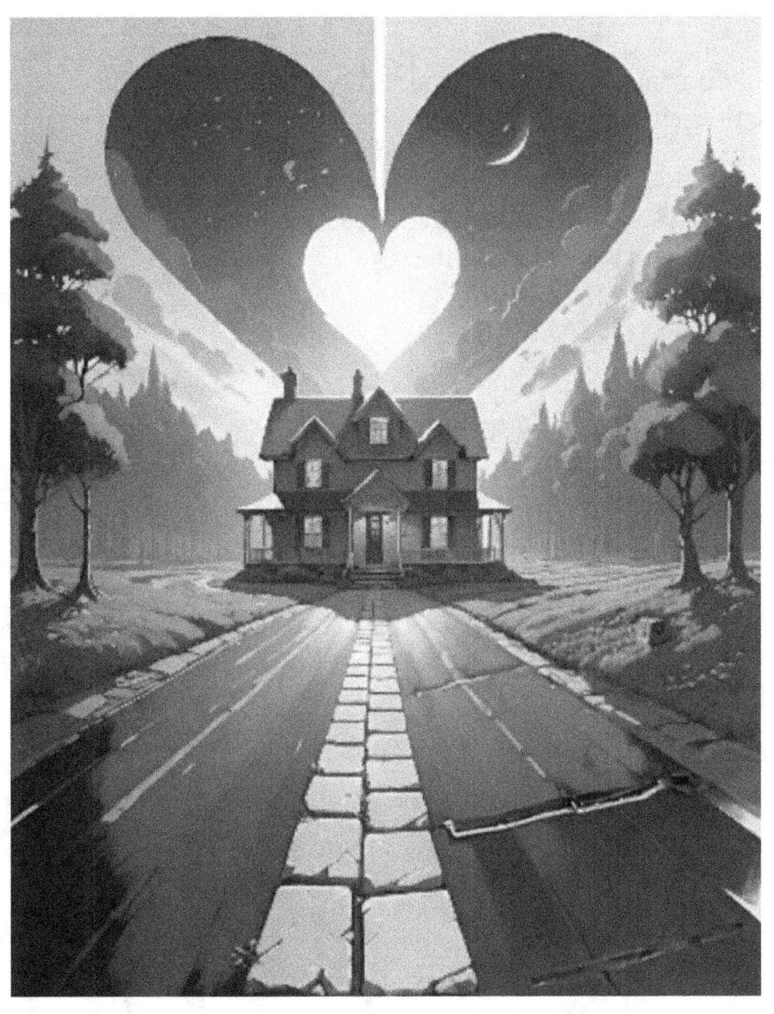

Home of the Brave Hearts

You and your sister traveling
different paths.

Two roads open yours paved with speed bumps
and grit.

Aesira's smooth and a little less fog
yet both reach the same sun
love's golden warmth
home

A place where you both bloom
wild and free each in your own way
both perfect

-N.B. Brignoni

FAMILY TIME NEVER ENOUGH
and I want a thousand years being your parent
a thousand years with you making you smile and laugh
holding you through everything.

-n.b. brignoni

two different worlds merge
i watched one daughter dance through fields of
milestones with ease showing me what the world
considers "normal" to be.

while the other dances on wheels and makes a miracle
come true.

as she finds her tempo in therapy rooms and hospitals
beds showing the world strong comes in many forms.

my two daughters in two different visions of the world
but in mine

it's two miracles
and no normal only
only appreciating the process of blooming.

two daughters in the same blessed gardens
of the infinite growing of a mama's heart.

-n.b brignoni

Mother's Hope

i love being a part of both worlds
merging them together

learning the ways
of your sister and yours

and i don't ever want to fall short
i hope I forever do a good job at making you
both feel like enough endlessly.

-n.b. brignoni

The Beginning of the Sisterly Bond

I can see it already the sisterly bond as Sira reaches for your hand.

She manages to grab it as you walk on the walker.

She caught you by suprise and you hold her hand with a funny expression of amazement tiny hands that made you smile and then break into a belly laugh giggle.

I stopped your sister before your hands made it into her mouth. She wanted to use your fingers as a teething toy. And you thought that was funny. So did I.

And it leaves me at awe happy tears for once and good family laugh.

-N.B. Brignoni

Mom's Search For Solace

B reathing in this bubble bath, a step towards healing a reset

R eflecting on the woman I see in the mirror a stranger to me

E xhausted, but still love being drained of my battery by my kids

A lien the shell of mine split, between the old life and the new one.

T o nurture myself in this steamy bath, a selfish act it seems,

H ow can I leave, as you sleep even for a fleeting dream?

E merging stronger, cleansing without tears learning to put the pieces to mend me whole, for you and your sister

I nhale the steam, exhale the fears, a mother's skin afresh.

N o longer broken hearted, maybe it's bending, adapting, growing with you.

O ut of the bath, back to your world, but carrying this serenity.

U nwinding the knots, breathing deep, a love that sets me free.

T o mend me whole nothing like the love of my children to revive me complete.

-N.B. Brignoni

My Eyes Scream

"Look," paramedics say, "Little one's happy over there."

Your sister with a smile in the corner unaware.

Normally, that sunny smile always warms my heart.

But this time was different, it was hot and cold bittersweet.

I knew, I was on borrowed time before she won't be oblivious at all.

Rather Instead, she'll see the fear in my eyes.

- N.B. Brignoni

It's Warmer with Two

daughters
i'm yours as i am hers
my two favorite girls
in this whole wide world

-n.b. brignoni

How do I explain seizures and sirens?
I don't want your tiny heart to hurt.

I want to wash away the fear with words but it's an
instinctive nature to be afraid as your sister has a seizure.

I want to teach you to be strong but you're so young you
shouldn't know the pain of worry yet.

So how do explains
seizure and sirens
when you sense it
something wrong
with your big sister
and the flush of worry
leads to chest pains.

-N.B. Brignoni

The Differences

and i, in silent watch nine-month-old
learn to stand at ease all on her own.

a milestone your sister hasn't learned

not used to this kind of parenting
a hands-off approach

where i witness milestones quickly
maybe i'm not ready.

I fear the day when the differences might sting.

My eldest you'll always be my normal
i love teaching you every step
waiting for my lessons
to click guiding your every way
ready to catch you
every fall

you've taught me
patience in the most beautiful way

even when training
falls through the cracks

it's okay will keep trying and
even if you don't get it i'll be there
waiting or appreciating what you can
because

no matter
the checkmarks
or empty boxes
you'll be loved no different
always perfectly you.

- n.b. brignoni

both girls
joys cure
or a heart's superhero
two daughters
become a light
in the dark
always showing me
the way
home

- n.b. brignoni

The Heart of a Mom Iron
I haven't
fallen apart
since you two
came along
I know this
is the strength
of a mom.

- n.b. brignoni

CHAPTER 15 THE GARDEN OF ATHENA

You'll Belong Everywhere

You were born different.
but still like a puzzle piece
finding its place
you fit
perfect

-N.B. Brignoni

Alternate Realities
If there was world
where perfection exists

I'd think of you still and i'd think of your
resilience, your strength, and your smile.

Even after everything we've been through all
the hospital visits and ambulance rushes.

I'd do it again
a thousand times
choose this path
choose you to be my daughter
i'd be your mom loud
and proud to be yours.

It's true what they say nobody's perfect
but if perfect is possible baby girl
i'd say it a billion times
perfect, is you.

you carry yourself
with such a light
i couldn't want a different
version of you

i'll always
love you as you are

-N.B. Brignoni

Warrior's Power

not many
like you on screens

no heroes
no leads
whom use
wheels that spin
stories of bravery
like you

little do they know
you're a firecracker
waiting to explode
being you is so different from
everyone else
that is a superpower in itself with a genetic code unique
being differently-abled

is beautiful a strength
you hold not a flaw

your resilent spirit shines
brighter than any Hollywood dream

you are just as deserving
as an abled-body

you belong on every screen
with a spotlight like a sun

that never dies

your worthy of it all my star.

this I know as you're
the best superhero i know

you saved me from Grief's hold

it could've been bad
i felt a magnetic pull from the depression
that was behind grief's door i was so close i could see a
blackhole through the crack that tried to suck me in.

but your hands
never let mine go
strongest superhero

i'll spend my life writing books about you so they can see
people like you should be superhero of the story.

-n.b. brignoni

our nest forever full
sweet
differently-abled
bird

geneticist
said your father
and I would never experience
empty nest syndrome

I never wanted
to see you leave
the nest anyways

you must stay
always with me
nestled close

forever
mine and his
a nest
never missing
a thing

and though my heart
aches for your freedom to fly like other
birds carelessly

i still hold on to hope that they are wrong
i see you older in my dreams a bird so pretty flying in
open skies and you had wings that defy.

- N.B. Brignoni

Baby Bird Must Not Leave The Nest

if it's not me giving you
wings

know you will fly with your family in open skies.

if it's not me giving you wings
know

it's your sisters, if it's not hers
it's your father's, if it's not his
it's your grandmother's, if it's not her
it's your grandfather's, if it's not him
it's your uncle's, if it's not him
it's your aunts, if it's not hers

you can count on wings
in your family to taste cotton clouds

you will always be loved in our nest
by them too not just me
you will never
be lonesome

perhaps this is the best possible
way to live life with people who love you

empty nest syndrome
is nothing i'd miss.

-n.b. brignoni

My Special Bloom

The world may follow a different beat.
But your rhythm's perfect, oh so sweet.

-N.B. Brignoni

Digital Dandelions
Rise, parents, rise,
and learn with me today.

I share my stories.
And I care to hear your tales.

Every missing petal
or extra holds magic
in every story.

If we share now
watch how each tale builds
another home with a lighthouse
stone by stone.

On screens where being different
finds light and strength.

Where all spirits soar, and wounded hearts find peace.

Together we could, dismantle limited walls.
Let love's garden increase.

A million blooms of dandelion seeds are
carried by winds, fulfilling hearts' needs.

We should stand together

for our little ones who fight.

In every struggle, we'll find
their strength and light.

And everytime we will rise
together at last.

- N.B. Brignoni

The Reason

maybe i have found it
the reason
fifty-four petals
plucked before your bloom
to share how even wildflowers
with missing pieces
bloom strong
roots deeper
for the loss
this is a strength
not a broken flaw

-n.b. brignoni

this is not the end
the greatest story
i could ever tell
is yours
Athena

and it's only
just begun
a story
you paint
with the stars

- n.b. brignoni

The last letter to myself
Dear past me, I bet you never could've thought the path
you traded in everything in for 2% universe road less
traveled full of miracles not the illusions of thorns and
blooms

Doesn't it feel good to not wear doubt like a second skin
To let go of grief

She is perfect you see her own wizardly series
with all the magic you and her keep making.

So proud you kept swimming through the tides. You kept
healing.

You didn't stop writing. Keep writing for them and you.
I've seen the books and they will cherish them forever.

A hint to the future the paint brush on her hand doesn't
stop.

The two percent path becomes more known and more
loved, thanks to you.

Don't ever stop writing to your daughter's they fall in love
with your stories. All the characters you make for them
become another friend for them to love and adore.
Sincerly, you, n.b. brignoni
in the future

I have a dream for my flower missing

petals
All the world will see
my daughter's laughter

her silence
still rings out
lights of the universe

she is liberated by the chain's
of medical odds

i have a dream
that her steps will be strong and steady
a march towards a future filled with hope
unburdened by the weight of limitations.

i have a dream
that her spirit will soar far passed the odds set
like an eagle on the wings of freedom

i have a dream for every child labeled
with boxes too check remember spirits can soar
beyond any checkmark on a page

and normal should remain a washing machine setting

our kids born different will dispell the labels
i have a dream
unfettered by the doubts of the world
only the world sees the sun
in her smile
the warmth it brings
they'll know it's needed

i have a dream of world
that'll love you
and see you
as your family always will

I have a dream of world
who sees you and the strength even in your
tiny frame

for you my little one carry
oceans on your back sometimes and still
shine like the moon
the sun
the stars
and everything
that lights
the very universe

it's you
Athena
the light
in all things
of my life

i have dream
the world will see too.

- n.b. brignoni

Epilogue

sweet girl
keep teaching
the world
that perfection
is found
in life's
imperfections
since the
moment you
were seed in womb
i have loved you
and i always thought
you were whole
perfect
missing petals
only means
you are more special
than you already were.

-n.b. brignoni

AFTERWORD

"The Missing Petals on Chromosome Four began as a journal of thoughts and feelings. On hard days, with music and late night writing, I tried to understand our situation in hospital rooms and therapy waiting areas. What started as a coping mechanism evolved into a narrative of love, resilience, and the unexpected beauty discovered while raising a child with Wolf-Hirschhorn Syndrome. Through these poems, I hope to illuminate the often Invisible struggles of navigating rare genetic disorders and remind others in similar situations that they are not alone. Together, we can craft stories of beauty amidst pain, transforming struggles into blossoming strengths. Every piece of our warriors' hearts is worth sharing."

ABOUT THE AUTHOR

"N.B. BRIGNONI is a parent and writer whose life was transformed by their child's diagnosis of Wolf-Hirschhorn Syndrome. Through poetry, they share their daughter's story and their unique perspective on the world, infused with love, challenge, and unexpected bliss. The author of The Missing Petals on Chromosome Four prefers to keep their identity private, letting the raw emotions and experiences within the poems speak for themselves. Each verse reveals the author's profound love and unwavering support for their child. The poems also narrate a journey of resilience, showcasing the author's capacity to find strength and hope amidst formidable challenges. If you wish to connect with the author, share your own story, or ask questions about rare illnesses, you can reach them at themissingpetals@gmail.com. They welcome your messages and look forward to hearing from you. The author aims to foster a safe space on their Instagram @TheMissingPetals_OnChromosome4, where individuals can unite to share warrior stories and ask questions. While maintaining their anonymity for now, they will continue to share their daughter's story through future books. The author sincerely hopes that the story inscribed in each verse of this poetry collection finds a place in your heart."

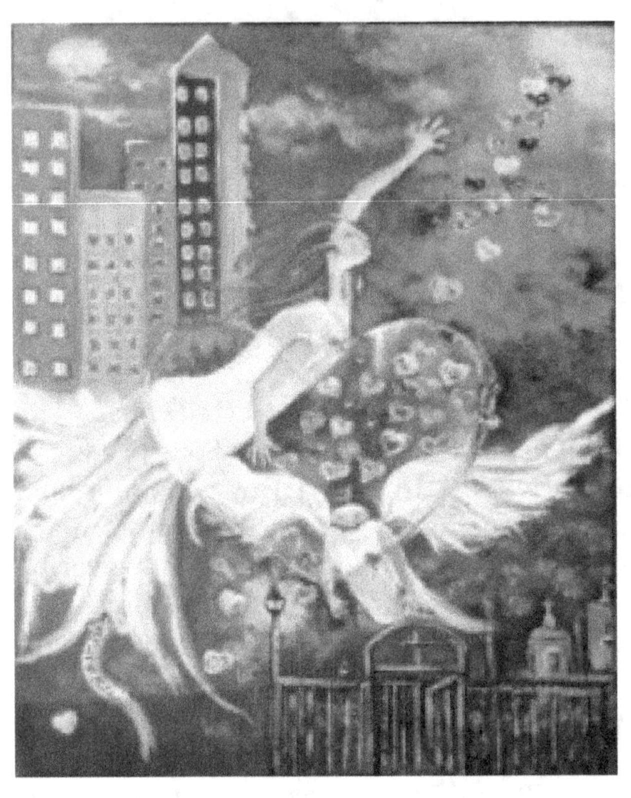

RESOURCES AND WEBSITES

1. Wolf-Hirschhorn Syndrome Foundation (www.4p-supportgroup.org): Provides information, support, and resources for families affected by WHS.
2. National Organization for Rare Disorders (NORD) (www.rarediseases.org): Offers comprehensive information on rare diseases, including WHS.
3. Global Genes (www.globalgenes.org): A leading rare disease patient advocacy organization.
4. Genetic and Rare Diseases Information Center (GARD) (rarediseases.info.nih.gov): Provides access to information about genetic and rare diseases.
5. The Epilepsy Foundation (www.epilepsy.com): Offers resources on epilepsy and seizure disorders.
6. American Physical Therapy Association (www.apta.org): Provides information on physical therapy and how to find a therapist.
7. American Occupational Therapy Association (www.aota.org): Offers resources on occupational therapy and its benefits.
8. American Speech-Language-Hearing Association (www.asha.org): Provides information on speech and language disorders and therapies.
9. Feeding Matters (www.feedingmatters.org): Offers resources and support for pediatric feeding disorders.
10. Parent to Parent USA (www.p2pusa.org): A national organization providing emotional and

informational support to families of children with special needs.

11. Complex Child (complexchild.org): An online magazine for families caring for children with special healthcare needs and disabilities.
12. Disabled World (www.disabled-world.com): Provides a wide range of disability and health information. Special Needs
13. Alliance (www.specialneedsalliance.org): A national organization of attorneys dedicated to the practice of disability and public benefits law.
14. Care.com Special Needs (www.care.com/special-needs): Offers resources and care options for families of children with special needs.
15. National Center for Learning Disabilities (www.ncld.org): Provides information and resources for learning disabilities and attention issues.
16. Rare Connect (www.rareconnect.org): An online platform for rare disease communities.
17. The Arc (www.thearc.org): Promotes and protects the human rights of people with intellectual and developmental disabilities.
18. National Down Syndrome Society (www.ndss.org): While focused on Down syndrome, offers resources applicable to many developmental disabilities.
19. Child Neurology Foundation (www.childneurologyfoundation.org): Provides resources for children with neurologic conditions.
20. Understood (www.understood.org): Provides resources for learning and attention issues.
21. Center Watch (www.centerwatch.com): Provides information on clinical trials.

22. EURORDIS - Rare Diseases Europe (www.eurordis.org): European alliance of patient organizations.
23. Simons Foundation Autism Research Initiative (SFARI) (www.sfari.org): Autism research news and resources.
24. National Center for Advancing Translational Sciences (ncats.nih.gov): Transforms the translational science process to get treatments to patients faster.
25. Patient Worthy (patientworthy.com): News and information for rare and genetic diseases.
26. RareShare (rareshare.org): Social hub for patients, families, and healthcare professionals affected by rare disorders.
27. MyGene2 (www.mygene2.org): Platform for sharing health information to accelerate research.
28. GeneDx (www.genedx.com): Genetic testing company with resources on various genetic conditions.
29. Syndromes Without A Name (SWAN) USA (www.swanusa.org): Support for families of children with undiagnosed medical conditions.
30. The Mighty (themighty.com): Digital health community platform for people facing health challenges and disabilities.

"Remember, while these resources offer valuable information, they are not a substitute for professional medical advice. Always consult with healthcare providers for personalized care and guidance."

1

BOOKS BY THIS AUTHOR

There is magic in missing petals. In a world where magic and reality intertwine, a forbidden love between the Greek god Hercules and a sorceress gives birth to you, Athena a child destined to bridge realms and wield unimaginable power. Yet your arrival is shadowed by a rare genetic disorder, casting a veil over your extraordinary destiny. As you grow, your parents navigate a realm filled with divine interventions, trickster gods, and the looming threat of the Twelve Labors. With each challenge, your resilience shines ever brighter, proving that even in the face of adversity, the human spirit nurtured by love and determination can transcend any limitation."